Schizo A

GW01081171

Carol E. Kelly

chipmunkapublishing
the mental health publisher

Carol E Kelly

Published by
Chipmunkapublishing
PO Box 6872
Brentwood
Essex CM13 1ZT
United Kingdom

http://www.chipmunkapublishing.com

Edited by Aleks Lech

ISBN   978-1-84991-686-8

Chipmunkapublishing   gratefully   acknowledge   the support of Arts Council England.

Chaper One Childhood

My early childhood was mostly happy with a normal birth at the Robinson Hospital in Ballymoney, County Antrim. I grew up in a little town named Garvagh in Co. Derry. From the word go, I was a dyed-in-the-wool tomboy, always getting into scrapes and adventures. I remember riding my tricycle round and round the square shaped elevated home, until one day I missed the corner and careered down the rockery into the hedge where an unsuspecting horse behind the greenery bolted like its life depended on it! I lay on my back seeing stars against the azure blue sky. My entire family were sitting having tea on the lawn on this particularly hot summer's day. To their chagrin there was a rather pregnant delay in serving up the sandwiches as I couldn't extract myself out of the thorny hedge.

Gradually they noticed that I was in difficulties and they then started to run to my rescue, but only after the startled horse had run off! One fine day, my eldest sister had the good sense to try and coerce me to jump off a three metre wall. I think I was a tender four years old. Thankfully I survived these daredevil shenanigans but it showed that even from a young age I had the heart of a lion. I was very courageous and could rise to any occasion.

My father was from Doagh, near Ballyclare and my mother hailed from Bovedy near Kilrea. They met in the Rathene Hospital, which is now a Nursing Home near the site of the old Coleraine Hospital, where he was a doctor and she was a nurse. Classic Mills and Boon material! After their marriage they settled in Garvagh, where my dad was the local GP.

During my early childhood, the family got a television (black and white set only in those days, the early 1960s). I never missed an occasion to bop around the living room to Top of the Pops! I loved to perform even back then.

As a tomboy tyke, climbing trees was a favourite adventure of mine and I used to love walking along the River Agivey with the family dog, a black Labrador called Prince. This beautiful dog was given to my father by a local millionaire. He was a wonderfully handsome and intelligent dog but he was so highly bred (the poor creature had a pedigree stretching back as long as your arm) he suffered from frequent fits. We weren't really allowed beyond the garden, but Prince and I used to trot together as happy as Larry for miles along the river. One day we got to a ford across the river. This was a cement road with pipes underneath for the water which had pretty strong currents. My beloved dog swam in the river as usual but got caught up in the currents towards the pipes. Well, he went in one pipe and a seemingly endless 5 minutes later, he came out the other side. I nearly dropped to my knees in thanks to God. When my dad died and we needed to move house, Prince had to go. My mum said he was happily living his days out on a farm. But whether this was an apocryphal tale I do not know to this day.

Meanwhile, turning our attention from canine to feline matters, the cat Sooty was a very prolific mother of dozens and dozens of kittens. Quite gruesomely, all of her offspring were drowned when very young by the gardener, under my mother's instructions. I watched one of these mass executions, always intrigued by what the part time gardener was doing. In a very traumatic event, while I was going through puberty the lust-crazed pervert gardener caught me in the dark and tried to rape me when I was a mere twelve years old. There was a fierce struggle and he broke my hymen and but there for the grace of God, I managed to flee his grasp. I never helped the gardener again.

Siblings-wise, I had two older sisters and a younger brother. My father was busy with his practice as a GP and my mum with her work as a nurse, assisting my father with his work. Unfortunately, my father suffered poor health and he had several heart attacks in his early 40's and by the age of 43 he was dead. My father had been held in very high esteem and he was very well regarded in his professional life. He was, in fact, secretary of the Northern Ireland British Medical Association. He enjoyed a drink and a smoke and refused point blank to give these vices up when he suffered the first of his heart attacks. My father began to lose his temper at home whenever he drank, and this turned into violence towards my long suffering mother and myself. One particularly harrowing memory I have is of one night when my father hit my mother on the chin. She desperately needed to go to casualty for stitches, but she could not bring herself to go in case the family secret was uncovered and my father, who had been described as, "Northern Ireland's best GP" was in anyway compromised. On another disturbing occasion, I was supposed to be studying for my Eleven Plus and my father leapt upon me where I was playing in the garden, dragged me indoors and started to thrash me. My mother made a desperate attempt at intervention and pulled down her underwear for him to beat her instead of me. This seemed to make him catch himself. In the end, my father died in his surgery, in front of my sister (it was half term). Despite the turbulent home life, I did not hate my father or despise him for the violence in the later years. He appreciated a drink and a smoke due to the pressures of his job. He could not give up these vices and he knew that they were going to kill him in the end. This is where all of his anger stemmed from.

The headmistress took us out of class one bleak cold February morning in 1969 and she told us that my father had sustained a fatal accident – I didn't know the meaning of the word fatal, but in my heart I knew something dreadful had happened.

I was allowed to go to the funeral service, but I was not permitted to go to the graveside. Instead I was packed off to a friend of the family's house. At this house their child of eight years age taunted me that I had lost my daddy but that she was lucky – she still had her daddy. I was ten years old at the time. My poor beleaguered brother had to go to the graveside in a boy's suit which he hated because he always had to wear the suit at funerals so it had unpleasant connotations for him.

My primary school years comprised of a very good education and also held a lot of fun times for me despite the existence back then of corporal punishment. It was also where my love of sport began. I played football as a goalkeeper at break time. One lunch time we broke a window with our football. I was terrified witless and I was also horrified that we were made to pay for the window (I was always saving up for the Sparky annual). These were hard times not long after rationing.

The various forms of corporal punishment were many and tortuous. Today they would be banned from use under United Nations Human Rights Law as Cruel and Unusual Punishment. There was the delightful cane with a hook on it, the edge of a ruler to the back of the knuckles or the little hairs pulled vigorously at the back of your neck - all in an average day's work at a normal Northern Irish primary school!

But maybe I am being too gloomy. There were great times to be had as well. The boys used to race the third of a pint milk in the little milk bottles when the headmistress wasn't looking. At this time in Northern Ireland education, milk was free for all children under eleven and it came in little glass third of a pint bottles. At home my bossy older sister consistently made a point of making me walk the plank in the game of pirates which we played off an old wooden structure. It was a wonder I didn't sustain some form of injury!

Trying to remember the good bits about my childhood is often difficult in light of the heartache with my father, but you can imagine now as an experienced and award winning Karaoke singer, I really did take singing and dancing to Top of the Pops into my hairbrush very seriously. My vocal talents were sufficiently developed for me to be chosen to sing the Christmas solo 'Away in a Manger' in the church my mother and father went to. I remained in choirs all of my childhood and teenage years. On one memorable occasion, I got to sing the middle verse of the carol 'Away in a Manger' and I messed it up, expecting an intro in the music as had always been done in practice. This pause nearly gave the organist and choirmaster a heart attack as it was a packed church for the Christmas Carol Service, but I had the chance to redeem myself in the evening service. Of course this was the 1950's and 60's and everyone went to church in those days.

As children, we were never allowed to sleep in on a Sunday morning and like youngsters all over Northern Ireland, Saturday night was always bath night. Friday nights were Girl Guides or Brownies. I was a keen camper because of my love for the great outdoors. Naturally I was a Girl Guide. In Garvagh I rose to the ranks of Sixer. Later when we moved to Portstewart, I was demoted to the ranks of ordinary Girl Guide again, because they did not know me as I was a 'blow in'. However, later in the Portstewart Girl Guides, I took up a position as a cub scout leader. We got to go away with the Guides and I proved to be a dab hand at pitching tents, digging latrines and lighting camp fires. However, one year we went to North Wales on a camping excursion and it rained all sodding week. We sang 'We ain't going to camp no more no more. We camped last year and the year before. We ain't going to camp no more'. In true Carry on Camping fashion, we were flooded out of the camp site and we had the joy of sleeping in a Scout Hall. The Girl Guides were an interfaith organisation, and due to this then pretty rare quirk in Northern Irish society, I got to make friends with Catholic girls. If it had not have been for the Girl Guides,

I mightn't have mixed socially with Catholic
university days.

My love of the outdoors had been cultivated by playing
in the huge garden that we were lucky to have in
Garvagh. As a small child I had built a little play hut at
the bottom of the garden where there were a dozen fir
trees. I constructed the hut with branches and twigs
from the trees; there were actually photographs taken of
myself outside the hut by my father when he was alive.
The intoxicating smell of fir was omnipresent in this hut.
Further down the garden I used to have exciting
adventures with the black Labrador dog. We frequently
crossed the river on the other side of the fence which
was an illicit thing for me to do, but I was never one to
heed the rules.

My father passed away in February 1969 and I had to sit
my first 11 plus paper around about October or
November in the same year. I woke up on the morning
of the first paper sick as the proverbial dog with nerves.
Despite my poor state of health, they let me go ahead
and sit the first paper, feeling like a nervous wreck. By
the time that the second exam rolled around, I was not
so nervous and the exam was a pushover. The

authorities must have noticed the big discrepancy between the two papers and later that December in 1969, they hauled me out of class and made me sit another paper, which presumably was a stand in for the first paper that my jitters had ruined.

Despite the hiccups, I passed my 11 plus and got into an 'A' stream at a highly academically esteemed all girls grammar school. However my initial euphoria and excitement was soon overshadowed by vicious psychological and physical bullying. The captain of the hockey team, an insufferable PE teacher's pet who couldn't subtract two from four and who also remained captain throughout my time at school, took an immediate dislike to me and took great pleasure in torturing me in various horrible ways. I was physically pushed around, regularly pushed out of the dinner queue and ostracised by nearly everyone at school. As the hockey captain this girl was very popular, or maybe it was through fear, but everyone seemed to follow her diabolical example.

One of the cruellest and most upsetting days at grammar school was at the Ulster School's Athletics Championships. This should have been the best day of my life as I managed to achieve a gold medal in discus, shot-put and relay, the only treble gold winner for the school. Quite a sporting feat. My arch nemesis, despite only coming fifth in her event – the javelin, was sent up to collect the Athletics Championship cup that I had won for the school. I was horrified to see her go up and accept all the glory, well aware of the pain and hurt I was feeling, as she snidely sneered at me whilst accepting the cup. I walked away feeling devastated, and I cried bitter tears.

Yet despite the bullying I learnt early on not to let it get to me, or perhaps I just became used to it. I soldiered on as best I could, enjoying and doing well in History, Geography and Maths, although I always found languages difficult to get to grips with – when it came to French it was a definite case of Je ne sais pas!

I did Art for three years and I showed great talent at it – coming top of the class at third year. But despite my Art teacher begging me to continue with it, I ventured into the world of Science subjects for O Level. Not a smart move. I failed dismally in Chemistry. "Why the heck did I drop Art?" I lamented to myself. As a consolation, I got an A grade in my beloved Geography. In fact, the highlight of my school years were the Geography field trips. One trip took me to the Yorkshire Dales, Ribblesdale, and a funny little town called Giggleswick – oh how we laughed! We found ourselves halfway down a mountain where we encountered rocks called erratics dumped by glaciers years ago.

Unfortunately I had a bad nose bleeds at these rocks and the teacher called them 'bloody nosed erratics'! But it was great to get away from the oppressive confines of the school. These trips also led to a few sneaky drinks parties – some fun at last. However, we were inevitably caught and heavily berated, but even the teachers got into the spirit, away from their normal habitat, and nothing was mentioned on our return.

Somehow, despite the regime at the grammar school and the pests who went out of their way to make my life misery, I obtained good enough grades in my A Levels – Geography, History, Biology – to attain a place at University in London.

Chapter Two Schizo as it was

In 1977, I crossed the waters to go to the South Bank University which was situated on the Wandsworth Road in London to study Estate Management. My ultimate ambition was to become an Estate Agent. I came from a family of high fliers – one of my older sisters was a doctor, my other sister was a nurse tutor and my brother speaks six different languages and works in management. On my father's side of the family, one of my cousins was Press Secretary to Mo Mowlam and Tony Blair. To top off this glittering roster, married to one of my cousins on my father's side is a judge.

When going to London I waited all day on a standby flight and finally arrived at my hostel in Kensington very late indeed. Nevertheless, I was up early the next morning to go to college, but unfortunately I ended up at the wrong tube stop and had to walk a fair distance to find the Wandsworth Road site. Not an auspicious start to my London adventure. The course was 95% male, as was the rest of the college, and it was very anti Irish as there had been a number of terrorist attacks in London and Birmingham around this time. Even the Pakistani and Indian communities were anti Irish and we could not fight back because we were white and we could not be seen to be standing up for ourselves against racism no matter where it came from. When it came to the social and racial pecking order, the Irish were the lowest of the low.

One Pakistani male student used to torture me for being a Paddy and also for being 'stupid'. Paddys or the Irish were always seen as being retarded, thick bricklayers and peasants, still with the donkey parked outside and a pig under their arms. The biggest 'ism' at South Bank was sexism, where 95% of the year was male and out of over 100 students there were only 5 girls.

Back at the boot campesque hostel in Kensington, I initially shared a room with a lovely girl called Jan. Though our friendship was strong, Jan hated the regime in the hostel. We had an ogre of a governess who was officially named Miss Weir but we gave her the monicker Miss Weirdo. The hostel had been strictly females only, but some male American students had been brought in that year and all sorts of shenanigans were going on upstairs in the rooms. There was always a sort of a curfew by which you could not get through the front door after 11pm. This was held strictly by Miss Weir, but it went by the board when the Americans were there.

Jan could not stand the strict regime and left for a flat in Brixton. As a result of this I became very lonely, but I got a room of my own on the top floor far away from anyone else my age. I made a few friends from the floors below but no one came to see me, so I withdrew into myself and spent a week not going out except to the bathroom. I didn't eat, sleep or speak. I just lay in bed staring at the four walls. This was the start of my drift into catatonia.

I was missed from college and Miss Weir called me to her apartment where she slipped me a Valium and ordered me to see the Welfare Officer at the college.

Along the way, I somehow got the thought into my head that I had to see Jan immediately. So I now, in a very dishevelled and disoriented state, travelled by tube to see her.

When I arrived, she immediately knew something was wrong just by looking at the very sight of me. She bathed me and took me to see the welfare officer at our college. As soon as we arrived at the South Bank's Welfare Office I imagined I was in a siege situation where the helicopters flying into nearby Battersea heliport were surrounding me. The workmen on the roof were really soldiers with guns instead of shovels. The sirens of the police cars were paddy wagons after me. In London, as I'm sure you know, there are always police sirens in the background, but I internalised this, thinking that they were all after me. The absolute terror and feeling of extreme paranoia that I was part of a vast conspiracy meant that I could not speak, and I must have looked both terrified and terrifying, and consequently very alarming in appearance to most people.

It was a Friday so Jan and I were sent home to get fish and chips in Brixton. No doctor had been called at this point. However, throughout the course of the weekend a doctor was sent for because I was so panicked and agitated I was acting like I was being frisked and standing against the wall so my torturers could search me. I went with the welfare officer, still not in any fit shape or form to speak, to the Maudsley Hospital. They begged me to sign a form which meant I was a voluntary patient. I eventually capitulated and for my sins, they put me in a cell overnight.

The next day, still devoid of the powers of speech, I was relocated to the Royal Bethlehem in Kent. It was one of the original Bedlams where the mad King George III had stayed in the late 1790's. Fortunately, progress had marched on since then and it was now an advanced research hospital.

I was to languish there for six unhappy weeks, but to jazz up the time I met a look-alike of George Bernard Shaw. He was always saying 'Oh what a game, what a game. Life is but a game.' Luckily for him, he got a bottle of Guinness every night and he also got his grey beard trimmed by the young nurses. George Bernard Shaw's look-alike was a real character. One time late at night (and I still wasn't talking at this point), he was reading his newspaper in a high backed chair with his back to us in the mixed sex living room. A young man came onto me as I sat there, and just as he was putting his hand on my knee, George Bernard piped up 'Oh what a game, what a game! It's a right fine game you two are having!' We were so embarrassed, and my mortified potential suitor fled out of the room like a bat out of hell.

Meanwhile my catatonic state was getting no better. The psychiatrists used to haul me in for an inquisition but I was silent. I began to mimic people's actions around me (a phenomenon known as echopraxia) which really got up everybody's noses. I mirrored the actions of other patients, nurses and psychiatrists without saying a word – even the cleaning ladies!

One time I was taken by taxi with a nurse to a hospital on the other side of London for a brain test. The nurse who took me I called Sister Luke. When I arrived at the hospital, I was appalled at the conditions that the patients were subject to. The sister was horrified as well at the state of the patients in this particular hospital, and we were both glad when we got back to Poppy in Kent where the Royal Bethlehem was based.

Occupational Therapy was much more fun in the Bethlehem than Gransha in Derry was to be, and I made some pretty nifty Christmas presents. On my release at the end of term the visiting psychiatrists called me an imbecileas as I still would not speak. This was in front of my mother who had come to rescue her daughter from the loonies. My mother protested that I had A Levels and that I was highly intelligent. Eventually my mum and myself managed to flee the institution through the underground to get the plane home. I was actually happier at travelling than my mother, who seemed to develop a bit of a nervous bladder problem and frequently had to go to the toilet on our journey.

Then came the Christmas vacation when I had to explain myself to my family and peers. It was made especially difficult when one of my older sisters, a medical student, came home. Pretty shortly after the holiday season, and despite my begging and protestations, I wound up in Gransha Psychiatric Hospital in the city of Derry, thanks to my sister's burgeoning medical know-it-all mind.

I spent four weeks there in that hell-hole they pretend is a hospital, and came out drugged up on Stelazine.

After the vicissitudes of Gransha, I started a part time job locally looking after pre-school children. I was the baby bouncer! The toughest baby bouncer in town! I separated three year olds who were going at it hell for leather in the play room.

They sat me in the playroom, gave me cups of tea and I fell asleep due to the sedating effects of the delightful drug known as Stelazine, until the noise of some child fighting with one another would wake me and I would separate them. Of course I also had to take them to the toilet and give them juice and biscuits but basically I was a baby bouncer!

By July 1978, I was given the all clear by one of those lovely psychiatrists to go back to London and retake my course in Estate Management. The following term I set off for Tooting to stay in a hostel which was a few tube stops away from the South Bank University. All throughout the course that year I snored away my time in Lectures, but I was not a completely inactive zombified slug. I was in training at night at Crystal Palace for athletics. The discus and shotput were my specialities, but I also liked to run as well. I used to jog around Tooting Bec Common. However, no amount of physical training could stop me from falling asleep all too easily in lectures. This was not my fault – it was not disinterest or apathy – I desperately wanted to pass my course, it was simply the effects of the medication. Unfortunately, by the end of the year I got hauled into the welfare office to be berated by the deputy welfare officer for failing my exams.

With every intention of staying in London, I was fortunate to get a job at the Wimbledon Tennis Championships. I really enjoyed working the two weeks there and soaking up all things tennis, being the sports nut that I am.

Then for reasons to this day I still do not understand, I was bundled off home by the welfare officer at South Bank University to what seemed to me to be a very bleak prospect of unemployment, no education and no future.

At home I had no transport to get to Ballymena and Antrim Athletics club to pursue my promising Athletics career. Yet despite all of these obstacles, I found an alternative route for my passion for sports and I immersed myself in all things to do with swimming. Being the perfectionist that I am, I couldn't be content to be just a good swimmer. I trained for and got my lifesaving awards, eventually becoming a lifesaving teacher and examiner and later a swimming teacher.

Due to my dedication and awards at swimming, I was always able to find various summer jobs in the following years with summer schemes, both as a lifeguard and a swimming teacher. One year I went to a beautiful scenic town in Northern Ireland and got a job as a Leisure Centre Attendant. I stayed with my other sister who was a nurse. At the facilities that I worked at, I was subject to severe bullying and sexual harassment. For instance, one time I was held under the water for a long time by a big burly bloke who later joined the RUC. This was at the height of the Troubles and sectarianism was rife. My liberal views about religion and politics were not tolerated back in those dark, dark days and I was subject to frequent taunting about them.

Fast forward to 1980. Whilst working as a Leisure Centre attendant I applied to go to the University of Ulster (Jordanstown) to study Sports studies (isn't that surprising?). I attained a high mark in my first year and as I was a popular student, I was voted class representative. During my time at Jordanstown I played volleyball for the university and we won the Northern Ireland Women's Volleyball League and were chosen to represent our province at international level in Dublin. I also played women's rugby for Jordanstown and we played Trinity College Dublin at College Park, beating them 22 points to 0. To our delight we were featured on the front page of the Irish Times in November 1980. So much for the imbecile the London doctors had pegged me for!

Whilst at the university I worked as a cleaner, cleaning the ceilings of the campus of dirt, dust and nicotine as a summer job. I started notorious bun fights in the canteen and generally had the time of my life. The work was hard but it paid the bills, and I was soon able to opt for a more pleasant job at a Leisure Centre closer to home, teaching swimming and volleyball.

After my jobs had finished and I was waiting for the academic year to begin, I went on a drinking binge in

Belfast. My friends at Jordanstown had persuaded me to come off my medication – bad idea. I ended up in a police station seeking help. I had entered the manic phase of bipolar disorder. During this time I went around engaging in a lot of strange behaviour, like pretending to be a child psychologist and going to Queen's University PE Centre pretending to be a Disability Officer. On another occasion, I visited a friend's house and put Stelazine in the Rice Krispies for reasons that are still unknown to me to this day.

When the summer was over I returned to Jordanstown in September and became increasingly manic, thinking I and everyone else in Jordanstown had contracted a very bad case of fleas. I even persuaded a psychologist whom I went to see that I actually did have fleas. She felt very uncomfortable with this prospect, as while I was in there I had claimed one of the little buggers had jumped onto her table. She referred me to the doctor. I got taken to Gransha by my uncle after a night when I disappeared on another drinking binge in Belfast. I ended up in a Police station polishing their rubber plants with Dobbins shoe wax. I thought I was making the place look more respectable.

There was still a sport's hall at this time in Gransha, there was also a film club at which I ironically saw High Anxiety with Mel Brooks in it. Remarkably for a psychiatric hospital, there was a dance once a week with a live band – usually a lamentable country and western band. So things weren't all bad. But it wasn't all sunshine, lollipops and rainbows.

There were the lock ups, the forced injections, the Largactil and the groundings for 'bad' behaviour. With the Largactil I put on a whopping four stone in weight, causing me a great deal of anguish since I was a dedicated athlete.

The university authorities had promised me I could return the following year to complete my course. All in all I spent six tortuous months in this mental hospital. I was diagnosed with manic depression, now familiar to most people as Bipolar disorder thanks to high profile cases in the media such as Catherine Zeta Jones. There was no mention at this point that I had Schizophrenia – but Bipolar was a definite diagnosis and label.

Gransha was a huge hospital with massive grounds including three rather picturesque lakes. The hospital had eight or ten villas for long term and lock up facilities.

I only knew of two villas outside of the acute clinics; thank heavens for small mercies! - Spruce for rehabilitation and Lilac for locking up female offenders, but there were many more. I was never in Lilac but I was in Spruce. Spruce was physically close to the exit and also mentally close as it was a rehabilitation unit.

Whilst I was in Gransha I was completely and utterly off the wall deluded. I got the notion into my head that I could make beer or cider with rotting apples, oranges, water and bread (bringing in the latter as it contains yeast) mixed up in hospital water jugs. Oh yes, I was going to run my own moonshine racket! At the same time I stole the master key to the clinic's front door. I may have been deluded to the eyeballs, but I was a very crafty mental patient!

Naturally, I got into big trouble for this and I got banned from going to the patient's weekly dance. It may have played country and western music, but I did enjoy twirling my toes on the dance floor so I was in fact quite bereft.

They also grounded me from walking in the grounds which really got my goat as I was a sportswoman and needed to keep fit. Even though I was banned from the hospital dance I chanced my luck and sneaked on to the bus to the dance hall anyway and later, as usually happens when mental patients try these illicit things, I got caught and was reprimanded once again.

The sum total of the care in Gransha consisted of queuing for tablets and eating indescribably awful meals. The psychiatrist was a virtual God and he not only had the power to force drugs down my throat, but he also had the power to ensure I was forcefully injected or grounded or let out for the weekend or released from hospital care. Rarely did the staff have any time for you, least of all the psychiatrist. He often saw patients in a ward round which was basically held in public for everyone to goggle at you like a freak show.

I remember waiting for six hours in the corridor for a psychiatrist. During this time I was afraid to go to the toilet in case I missed him. This is an example of the power they had over us.

In the middle of one of my stays at Gransha the psychiatrist released me for the weekend to go to an athletics meeting where I won one gold and one silver medal at the Ulster Sport's Council Athletics Championship in the Discus and the Shot Putt.

Nowadays there are no sports halls, no film clubs and no dances. There are fewer and fewer big hospitals that have these facilities; most long term patients are in the community.

The number of mental health care workers has decreased in the community. There are fewer Community Psychiatric Nurses and I'm told there is a two year waiting list to see a psychiatric social worker in my trust area. So much for community care. The government have stripped the assets of our hospitals and they have not replaced it with anything much to show for the millions of pounds they have gained.

Government policy is to take as much out of mental health hospitals and grounds as they can, thereby pushing vulnerable people onto the streets and not providing care for them in the community.

Psychiatrists, CPN's and psychiatric social workers can do little to stop this demise. They can only watch as their resources dwindle and their budget gets tighter and tighter. Apart from the government, the only ones making a profit are the pharmaceutical companies selling drugs by wining and dining the doctors, sending their representatives to cajole doctors into buying into the medical model rather than the social model of psychiatry. The medical model of psychiatry consists basically of prescribed drugs whereas the social model consists of talking therapy, like cognitive behavioural therapy. The government does not want the pharmaceutical industry not to gain money from their drugs so they favour the medical model.

Getting away from politics and going back to my time at Gransha, during my time in hospital I was a bit of a hippy or perhaps it's closer to the mark to say tramp! Caring little for my appearance, I dressed down rather than up but I was totally elated whilst doing so. I think other patients were afraid of me because I looked so down-at-heel, but I didn't give a fig because I was in such a good mood.

I collected twigs and leaves and branches from my walks in the woods beside one of the lakes. I filled my cell with wild flowers and twigs, and on the walls I had the newspaper cuttings of the prowess of my sporting days. This elation lasted several months, and I had a colleague in the cell beside me with whom I used to go walking to collect these various trappings of nature.

Meanwhile my appetite for food was vastly increased, being on the anti psychotic drug Largactil. At one particularly gut-busting sitting I remember that I ate two dinners and three puddings!

I rocketed from 11 stone to over 17 stone in a period of three months. None of my clothes fitted me so I was left slopping around in tracksuit bottoms and dodgy jumpers. The grounds of the hospital were fantastic though, with paths leading to beautiful woods and lakes and a working farm for the long term residents.

In O.T. (Occupational Therapy) you could sew or knit or paint. I wanted to learn how to make frames for pictures, but that seemed to be strictly a male occupation. Some things the women were allowed to do and some things the men could do. It was highly sexist. You were only allowed to attend O.T. if you were well enough. I mainly crocheted babies' blankets for my increasing number of nephews and nieces. Often these blankets became comfort blankets for them and they would not go to sleep as infants without them.

Eventually my elation decreased and I crashed down into a state of depression. The domestics cleaned out my room and took all the forlorn looking twigs away and my newspaper cuttings were binned. The cell got back to its clinical appearance and all my lovely flowers were gone.

In the Halls of Residence at Jordanstown after my first stay at Gransha, I wrote a poem entitled 'Waiting in the Lobby' which has become my signature poem for which I am most famous. It is on the internet – on You Tube in a short film made by Patrick Trojlan called 'Considering Carol' in which I give a performance of the poem. This short film won an award from Northern Ireland Skillset Media Academy in 2010 for best Postgraduate Project. The poem describes my feelings upon entering and leaving psychiatric hospitals

Waiting in the Lobby:

Waiting in the lobby of the hospital,

All my friends have left me,

Even Steve and Sal.

Only left with my emotions,

Which they tell me, lie to me,

They tell or they suggest that I am not normal, and yet I feel normal.

Oh no – just a little confused, just a little bemused at what is going on.

Doctors, nurses, staff seem to wait behind, out of sight but not out of mind.

They seem to wait for my next reaction,

For my next attraction to another human communication.

Communication, that is what is lacking, that is what they are attacking.

Even with all my courage, I cannot eat, I cannot speak, and even left beside me

The brown-grey liquid called 'Hot Chocolate', which is not touched.

Everyone is so nice here, the staff that is.

All my other comrades seem to laugh at me.

All the shades of black humour which surround this condition,

The omission of reality.

For the cold, hard world outside, that once opened the door for me,

Has seen me lying on the floor, stripped naked of my self respect,

The blatant image that reality was too hard, and too coarse for my finer feelings.

That is what it was like, yes that is what it was like.

So now I find, a brave world, good

But fair,Where kindness and caring are not just part of somebody's working day,

Measured out to each lost cause, to help them on their way.

No, it's not like that any more,

Now when I try at something, it is not false praise that I get,

Though praise is less than it once was, it is at least meaningful.

Not dressed up in a uniform like an army dame.

The world is kinder to me now,

And the reality which I have is not questioned at every turn,

Is not something which I have to learn.

The person which I find each day is me –

A somewhat shy, somewhat quiet thinker

In a non-thinking world.

This is why I wrote this, for you to think,

For you to think, 'Thank God I have my sanity'

Chapter 3 My Sporting Life

From a very early age I was a highly active child. Today I would be described as ADHD with a few other disorders thrown in and probably prescribed Ritalin to boot! More often than not I had some war wounds from my antics, mostly from falling out of trees and some from vicious scrapes with my brother. However, I have a very vivid memory of when I first discovered the joys of sport. I was nine years old and the local under twelves were practising at the nearby football pitch. I desperately wanted to play as I had kicked a ball about a bit and I knew I was just as good as most of the boys. But in the sixties, in rural Northern Ireland, girl football teams did not exist, and so from an early age I understood the barriers that existed for me as a girl. Little did I know then that I would spend a large part of my adult life fighting and crusading against discrimination of all shapes and sizes. However, on this Saturday morning as I stood forlornly at the sidelines I was called over by the coach. He proceeded to tell me I could play with the lads as they were a player short. I stared in disbelief, jaw hanging; I was stunned. Thankfully I quickly regained my composure, and shocked the coach by grabbing him around the legs in gratitude! I ran onto the pitch – all guns blazing, I had a lot to prove. I didn't let myself or the team down, even managing a sliding tackle! Afterwards I received lots of praise from the coach on how well I'd played. I basked in the adulation and recognition, at last I felt I had a real talent. I was every bit as good as the best male players. Of course it was to be a short lived triumph. The hard reality was that regardless of how good I played as a female I would never be allowed on the team. Although painful as this was, it also proved to be an important lesson in the ways of the world. At this young age I recognised discrimination and I knew it was wrong. Despite this it certainly signified the start of my sporting life. After that football match I knew I wanted to have that feeling of exhilaration again and compete in as many sports as possible.

From the age of seven I was a member of the local Tennis Club in Garvagh. This was a sport I excelled in and I was able to compete in this game without barriers because of my sex. With the club just down the road, I was to be found most summer evenings there; the club was only closed on a Sunday. I played in many tournaments and I was even asked to organise one by the tennis coach who was also my headmistress. I was thrilled to be chosen for this important task, however being only twelve I seized the chance to make sure that I played in every game, whilst others sat on the sidelines waiting for their turn! I don't think it endeared me to the other members – in fact, thirty years later, I bumped into a friend from those days, who reminded me of what I'd done and insisted on a grudge match! At Grammar School I was forced to choose between tennis and athletics and I decided to choose athletics, and that was the end of my competitive tennis career. However, years later whilst studying in London I applied to work at Wimbledon Lawn Tennis Championships. To my delight I was chosen and for a lifelong tennis fan, this was heaven! I watched the mighty Navratalova defeat Chris Evert Lloyd. I also met Navratalova's mother who had been allowed out of Communist Czechoslovakia for the first time to see her daughter play. This was the first time they had seen each other since Navratalova had defected to the US. As John McEnroe was being beaten by one of the Gulockson twins I happened to be standing next to a very upset NBC reporter who was covering the match. It was a great thrill to be witness to these important events whilst serving the traditional strawberries and cream! Each morning I had to travel from the other side of London. I was often late but somehow managed to get away with it - it must have been the Irish charm! As a country girl this was all very new. I got a taste for the finer things in life. I developed a love for iced coffees, something I'd never heard of. But it was an amazing experience to be in amongst the world's elite tennis players and a long way from the Garvagh Tennis Club!

When I went to Grammar school the world of sport really opened up to me. Sports were strongly encouraged and I excelled at quite a few while I was there. I did tennis, hockey and athletics. I particularly enjoyed hockey, probably because of the camaraderie of the other girls. I was on the under fourteen A team. The team had a lot of success, winning county championships regularly. Unfortunately I sustained a knee injury and was dropped from the first eleven. At the time I felt my injury was just the excuse my coach was looking for. The team Captain had taken a real dislike to me, for reasons I still don't know. And the coach, for reasons unknown, seemed to have a real soft spot for the team captain! So as the captain had it in for me so did the coach, and I was conveniently dropped. My revenge was to join the second eleven team and go on to have much more success than the first team. We won every competition we played in that year!

At the age of fourteen I began athletics and showed most promise in the discus, shot putt and relay. I won the Ulster School Girls Championship for the school in all three disciplines. But my victory turned sour when at the awards ceremony on the Malone Road in Belfast, my nemesis the hockey team captain went up to accept the prize that I had won for the school. I walked away crying bitter tears of humiliation...

When I went to Jordanstown University I began to play volleyball. I was a substitute in the team, but the volleyball game has many substitutions. Bringing me on was always a gamble because, typically of a manic depressive, I was either brilliant or terrible! But nevertheless we managed to win the Northern Ireland Championships and we got selected to the European Championships which were held in Dublin. However, there were riots in Dublin that year – 1981, in protest for the Hunger Strikers, many of which turned violent, and a few teams pulled out, including England and Germany. At another tournament in Dublin we were left with no accommodation. Both the male and female teams, about twenty in all, were forced to share a very cramped two up two down, with one outside toilet. Needless to say our performance in our matches the following day wasn't great by any stretch of the imagination! What I enjoyed most about my time playing volleyball was our trips around the country - lots of girls on a minibus ensured high jinks and lots of laughs. I'll always remember when we had to get the bus to stop to let us off to relieve ourselves, as a few drinks were taken to celebrate a win. The bus stopped late at night somewhere around the border in South Armagh. Squatting in a field, next thing we knew we were surrounded by British soldiers and literally caught with our pants down! Though I'm sure that was a pleasant surprise for soldiers on cold wet night in South Armagh. Peeing at the side of the road was a constant source of fun and danger with all sorts of high fences being scaled in order to preserve some form of dignity!

Rugby was another sport that I really enjoyed at Jordanstown. My height and strength were a great advantage. I played second row, one of the forwards. Again this sport took me all over Ireland playing matches. One of our great achievements was going down to Dublin to play Trinity College on College Park.

During the match I managed to get a run with the ball and get through five tackles. But just before the try line I came up against Big Christine, an American football player, who threw me to the ground like a rag doll and I lost the ball. However we won convincingly 22 – 0 and the following day our picture adorned the front page of The Irish Times. Rugby being rugby we knew how to celebrate, and drinking games were an important part of the culture. One particular night in the environs of Augher, Clougher and Fivemiletown I was up against a girl to down a pint in the fastest time. This girl had the very special skill of being able to pour a pint straight down her neck. Because she opened her gullet and poured it straight down in seconds flat I had had to pour nearly a full pint over my head. I was in some state, soaked head to toe and stinking of beer. I dreaded returning home; my poor mother was not impressed with this drunken mess that arrived back on her doorstep.

I became very passionate about rugby and was loath to stop playing. So when I went to The University of Ulster Coleraine Campus and discovered they had no team, I founded one. I was also Captain of the team. At our first tournament we were trounced by a visiting Warwick University team. At this stage I had turned thirty and was considerably older than the other players. I injured my knee badly in the game. But I was determined to continue playing. The following year we invited Warwick over for another tournament and this time we managed to defeat them by a single try. We won a Tyrone Crystal Rugby ball, which was tossed around the changing room and by some miracle wasn't dropped.

Sadly after university my rugby career came to an end but I remain a passionate supporter of rugby in the safety of my front room!

Swimming is a sport that I discovered after my school years. As a child living near the coast most summers were spent swimming in the sea. But it was always purely for fun and involved a lot of splashing about, and my technique was terrible. Swimming changed for me when I was home from university one summer and a friend offered to show me some techniques to improve my swimming. And improve I did! I realised with the proper technique I was quite a strong swimmer. I had very good upper body strength from my years of discus and shot putt. Encouraged by my progress, my friend and I did a life saving course. From there I continued to gain more swimming exams, and qualified as a swimming teacher and gained an examiner qualification from The Royal Life Saving Society. Swimming had become a real passion for me and I enjoyed gaining more experience which I was then able to pass on to others.

And the truth is that swimming had saved my life during a very difficult time. As a result of my illness I was asked to leave my degree course at Jordanstown. I was then hospitalised for a year. Upon leaving hospital I knew I wanted to pursue more swimming qualifications; it had become my lifeline during this bleak time. I was able to gain experience teaching through local summer schemes, where I taught kids of all ages swimming. I thoroughly enjoyed it, and it gave me back my confidence, which had received such a battering from the enforced exile from the Sports Studies degree at the university. I felt badly let down by them and very angry at their lack of understanding in dealing with my illness. By 1986 I had gained enough experience to take up a position with Belfast City Council as a peripatetic swimming teacher, serving six different leisure centres around the city. This was at the height of the troubles but I loved this job, and the new start it represented for me.

The backdrop to my new found mental stability and purpose was a very unstable and violent Belfast. I lived in a flat in the Ballysillan estate, one of the most troubled hot spots, in Loyalist North Belfast. At night shots would ring out, followed by the sirens and chaos. A friend's flat was burnt out because of a previous career in the Security Forces. That night I waited anxiously for him to come home, or what was left of him, from a particularly troubled night in the city. Whilst waiting I wrote this poem.

Waiting
Tearing myself in two
It is because of you
Agony on agony
The ecstasy to come.

Ever ever waiting
Contemplating
The things we might have done
But war, this war
Got in the way.

Your every move frustrated

Never, never nearer
Always far away
So holding you much dearer
You've gone amiss, astray.

And so I'm left awaiting
The outcome of it all.
Perhaps the news on North Belfast
Will hear your dying call.

Thankfully my friend returned home safely that night. Unfortunately it was to discover his flat burnt out. He came to stay with his mother who lived in the flat beside me.

Another night I saw a dead girl being dragged past my front door. Most people during the Troubles developed a coping mechanism to deal with the horror around them. We blocked it out and kept going; what was the alternative? I was to discover later in my MA dissertation, as the homicide rate goes up the rate of suicide goes down and inversely so. The existence of an external enemy means we are less likely to develop an internal enemy and therefore depression. Our innate survival instinct was very strong in the face of all this violence. How healthy this was for our society is another question.

Nevertheless, life with the backdrop of the Troubles went on. In the academic year 1986-87, I was successfully employed as a swimming teacher. I absolutely adored the work, but once again my mental health woes reared their ugly head considerably exacerbated by the Troubles. I was in the Mater Hospital over the summer in 1987. For being a psychiatric ward, it ranked rather high on the scale of decency – the nurses were very efficient and kindly. It was such a breeze, I came up with a little saying 'It doesn't really matter, you are only in the Mater'. However, yet again I came face to face with an old enemy called Largactil, which is an antipsychotic medication. It made me gain four stones at a breathtaking pace. Whenever I was discharged and returned to work in September 1987 I was overweight and yawning in the chlorine soaked heat of the swimming pools. My boss asked me to sign a form. I didn't have a clue what it was, but he was rather eager that I sign it. It turned out to be the termination of my contract. My sporting adventures in the Big Smoke were over and I returned home in a state of abject defeat, deprived of what I loved doing most – sport.

However, you can't keep a good sportswoman down for long. In 1988, I was a babysitter for a Judo coach and his wife and children and he persuaded me to come along to Judo training. Initially I didn't like it much, as one of the moves was to smother your opponent, and they didn't talk of contests – they spoke of fights. This led to me having a love/hate relationship with Judo. As a team (University of Ulster Coleraine Campus) we entered the Northern Ireland Judo championships. I had to face the Commonwealth champion who also was an Olympian. In judo if you don't make a move in so many seconds, you get penalised. I was afraid of being penalised, so I made a move. I lasted 17 seconds against the champion and was upended on my back. I was so grateful not to be injured, I shook her hand and was called back to bow, Japanese style. This was a Queen's University PE Centre. I ended up winning the Silver medal. That was the height of my Judo career!

Carol E Kelly

Chapter Four Swimming not Drowning

I started my lifeguard and swimming career as a beach guard on East Strand, Portrush and also Downhill Beach. All was quiet until one day on the East Strand there was an off shore breeze and an incoming tide and loads of lilos and floats in the water. Way outside of my flagged area a little 10 year old boy swam after a rubber tyre. He got into difficulties and his father, who could not swim, desperately tried to go after him in a futile attempt to rescue him. I ran 600 yards as I was at the nearest flag and I managed to save the son, only to realise the father was still in the water. I put the son in the recovery position. The tide was still coming in. I did a search and rescue for the father, but he was nowhere to be seen. The current began to drag me under too. We nearly had another fatality. I returned to the son, the tide was lapping at his feet, I lifted him up gently and placed him away from the water. He was to spend 48 hours in intensive care. The father's dead body was washed up. I tried to resuscitate it but I could not clear the air way. An ambulance arrived and took over. A helicopter was sent out and offshore rescue. It was too late for the father – he had died. Luckily the son survived. His mother was understandably distraught. I got a citation in the inquest

"The lifeguard did all she could do under the circumstances and showed no little courage in what she did." This was published in the local press and people mistook 'no little' for 'very little' when in fact it meant the exact opposite – great courage. One particular lifeguard gave me a hard time about it in the pub. The following day we had nine rescues on the one day in similar conditions – off shore wind and incoming tide. Being a beach guard is certainly not an easy glamorous job, the way that they portrayed it in Bay Watch!

My career as a swimming teacher and lifesaving instructor really came into full blossom when I worked 29 hours a week for Belfast City Council as a swimming teacher. The job required me to be a peripatetic swimming teacher which meant I worked all over Belfast. I worked in Shankill Leisure Centre, the Falls swimming centre, the Anderstown Leisure centre and the Grove Baths. In fact, pretty much any swimming pool owned by Belfast City Council. I used to ride my bicycle between them, bravely venturing through various Peace lines at the height of the conflict.

When I first arrived in Belfast, I was homeless but within days the Shankill Road Mission put me up because my work was based at the Shankill Leisure Centre. Until the Housing Executive could give me a flat I stayed with a stranger called Tommy. When I arrived at Tommy's two up two down house on the Shankill Road, Tommy opened the door to me with his belt undone and thus his trousers hanging off. This wasn't a very auspicious introduction, but nevertheless he put me up for a week without touching me in any inappropriate way.

When I finally got a NIHE flat it was in Ballysillan. Now there was the infamous Shankill Road butcher operating at this time (1986) but there was also the notorious Ballysillan butcher who turned out to be just down the street from me. It was at the height of the troubles in this area but I had a very helpful and decent neighbour downstairs. She used to give me a cup of tea and a piece which turned out to be a slice of bread and butter, every afternoon when I finished work.

I worked every day until 3pm with the schools, and then I taught night swimming classes with both children and adult classes all over Belfast. Whilst teaching adults in the Falls Baths, the facilities actually still had bath tubs for workers and men especially still used those bath tubs. I met a few characters in the adult classes in the

Falls and the Grove baths. I once asked an elderly lady 'Why did you never get married in your lifetime?'. She said it was because 'The Obtainable was not Desirable and the Desirable was not Obtainable'. I thought this was a very good answer and wrote a poem about it. One time when I went out for a drink on my own in Kelly's Cellars I got mistaken for an undercover policewomen and one bloke tired to lure me back to Poleglass, an estate in the west of Belfast. I managed to escape home in a taxi. I can assure you I was absolutely petrified as these were very scary times. Thus the poem the Obtainable was not Desirable.

The Obtainable was not Desirable

Far away now he wooed me,
With the same old stories
Of love and involvement.
His prejudices stuck out a mile.
The milk of human kindness
Was not to be found there.
Far away now,
I can get back on the fence,
Love which came and love which
I chose to let go

Far from the hazards
Of bitter city life,
Now on the train
I see the lambs and the trees
Getting greener for another
Short summer, with a long time
To avoid the Marching season

Other poems I wrote during my stay in Belfast were Waiting and a Rainy Day in Belfast. One time my neighbours son's flat got burnt out not far away from where I lived. We were also in perpetual fear of his life, coming as he did back from work on the other side of the city on a troubled night. I was very fond of him and so I wrote this;-

Waiting

Tearing myself in two, it is because of you.
Agony on agony, the ecstasy to come.
Ever, ever waiting contemplating
The things we might have done
But War this War got in the way,
Your every move frustrated

Never, never nearer
Always far away
So holding you much dearer
You've gone amiss, astray
And so I'm left awaiting
The outcome of it all,
Perhaps the news on North Belfast
Will hear your dying call.

Being bipolar and Schizoaffective I was very vulnerable to the troubled environment around myself and the conflict considerably exacerbated my illness. I only lasted a full school year miraculously unaffected, but finally in June the paranoia took over and I admitted myself to Flat One, the Mater Hospital. This was OK because I was in the psychiatric ward of a General Hospital, so it didn't seem as stigmatised as being in a full blown mental hospital. I used to help the other patients by saying 'It doesn't really matter because we're only in the Mater'. That is it could have been worse and we could be in the 'Burn' (which stood for Purdysburn, now Knockbracken Healthcare Park) and all the stigma surrounding that.

During my stay in the Mater, the height of Summer 1987 and the 12th July, there was a very elderly lady in the bed beside me. She was known as Cissy. She had multiple problems; only one was psychiatric. I don't know if she had cancer as well or some other debilitating illness, but Cissy had difficulties communicating. However I soon learnt that if she made a noise she probably wanted to go to the toilet. Getting her to the loo was one thing but getting her to go to the loo was quite another, so we used to turn the taps on in the bathroom, the noise of which would make her go. Thus the poem Ode to Cissy.

Ode to Cissy

There is a very subtle line here
This is where the lost come to rest
The followers of age and confusion
Confused by the world outside
They also wonder why their whisperings
To loved ones are not heard.
Senile and cynical,
With lost hopes and forgotten dreams
Trying to rebuild the old,
Or replace the new.
We laugh at their innocence at such an age.

"No one will see you now Cissy,

You can pull up your skirt."

The command gently given as

The commode on wheels pulls up –

Just a symbol of the modern age.

Cissy tries to fathom how she can go to the toilet, and be in a wheelchair at the same time.

"Don't worry Cissy, the taps in the bathroom

Are turned on full, just for you".

Strong is the ageing mind, when it comes to when

And where one should go to the toilet.

"Oh Cissy, please don't be perturbed,

This is where the lost tend to go."

The staff kept me in the dark when Cissy was taken to a Nursing Home and I was left without my constant companion over the 12th July holidays, cast to the banging of the drums, and feeling isolated in Belfast. There was a very good occupational therapist there and we had great fun in role play. There were in fact quite a number of good nursing staff compared to other psychiatric units, but I was itching to get back to work.

While I was in the ward at the Mater, they put me on a drug called Largactil. Largactil is an antipsychotic – it is in fact the first one ever invented. It has numerous unpleasant side effects – it gave me a huge appetite and it consequently made me put on lots of weight.

When I finally cycled back to work from a shared house off the Ormeau Road I was three to four stone overweight. Thank you once more Largactil!

My manager at work hounded me to see if I was making any mistakes due to my obesity. I did do a lot of yawning in the new classes due to the combination of the heat of the swimming pools and also my medication. One day the coaching coordinator my boss came along with some papers which he said I had to sign. They were unbeknownst to me, my resignation papers – there was I thinking they were there to renew my contract. Anyway I signed them and only afterwards did he say Belfast City Council were releasing me, I had to pack up and go home to my mother with my bicycle.

I spent the next two years making new friends at home and going to the local Arts Centre to do pottery, creative writing and Art. Meanwhile my mother started to have strokes T.E.A. I increasingly had to nurse her through this traumatic time. The attacks left her paralysed down both sides and eventually confined to a wheelchair, to our dismay. It started with loss of balance and pins and needles feelings down her arms. One time I left her in the garden, a place that she loved, and I went down to take a message to the local shop. Unfortunately it started raining cats and dogs and I was infuriatingly delayed at the shop. With her lack of balance my mother could not get back to the bungalow so she got drenched. She was hiding for shelter under a bush when I got back so I rescued her from this indignity and gave her a hot bath.

This disability continued in the ongoing years and she became increasingly
much more debilitated as she got older, but she was only 60 when she retired from her work as an occupational nurse. I remember going in to help her at work, but she had to leave as she was too debilitated. Caring for my mother was not easy; this role reversal did not sit easy with either of us. I found it physically and mentally draining and eventually we both had to accept that she needed to go into a Nursing Home.

A Tear from Her Eye

I wiped a tear from her eye,
She could not wipe the tear away herself,
She who had borne me,
She who had wiped away my first tear.
I swept the water from her face,
And kissed her
As I always kissed my mother.
We ate; my meal went cold,
As she had first fed me,
the babe in her arms,
Had drank her milk
And rose to lift her now.
A dead weight. Not dead spirit,
But very much alive.
I carried her to the car which she can no longer drive.
And thought of how
She visited me as I visit her now,
In an institution.
I went home and cried,
No one was there to wipe away my tears.
I left her in the home,
For her food to be fed to her.
I cried as I thought of the love

She had given,
And I in my mania had lost,
But regained in my mum today.

I was very fortunate to have been able to share this poem with my mother before she died. I remember very clearly that day. A family friend was visiting also, and when I'd finished the poem all three of us had a good cry!

My mother remained in the Nursing Home until she died in 1998 at the age of 71 years, when pneumonia, the old people's friend, took her away. One day whilst leaving her in the nursing home my sister and I walked the beach but had forgotten our mobile phones. Thus the poem 'Walking the Strand'.

Walking the Strand

I call to my sister
Let's go home.
Our mother is dying
And I'll be alone.

She lay there sleeping
As we walked the beach.
Afraid of her dying
And us out of reach.

Together
We buried her
Hand in hand
The coffin was lowered

I still walk the strand.

Whilst my mother was still alive she saw me off to a university degree for the third time. This time to the local University of Ulster at Coleraine where I did a Combined Humanities degree, major history, minor geography. I unfortunately failed my first year but I passed at the resits and did enough to get a reasonable degree whilst founding and captaining the university rugby team. The team went from strength to strength until our male coach went off with all our money. We even managed to snare a broadcast on Radio Ulster due to our efforts and success. To top it all off, we won a crystal rugby ball at a tournament which our dastardly male coach kept. These years at the University of Ulster at Coleraine saw me finally achieve my academic and social goals that I had fought for for many years. The illness that had scuppered my earlier attempts was kept at bay. However, I was always aware of its presence and power to wreak possible havoc in the future.

Chapter Five Out and About

For what seemed like many years, but which actually amounted to five in all, I had the good fortune to work on some of the Causeway Coast's most scenic attractions. I was employed to recruit membership for a large conservation charity. I worked at Carrick-a-Rede Rope bridge, Whitepark Bay, The Giant's Causeway, Downhill and Portstewart Strand. These were all some of the most beautiful places in Ireland – North or South - to work, especially as it was during the summer season, and from memory anyway, the sun shone a lot! It was quite a physically demanding job, a lot of walking was involved and every day was spent outside. It did wonders for my fitness levels and my complexion!

Downhill was my most memorable posting as I worked there for four summers straight. My days were spent walking around this magnificent estate from the The Musseden Temple, (a folly built by The Bishop of Derry, who was also Earl of Bristol, for his niece, with whom he was in love – he called her cheriecousine!) perched precariously on the cliff top with its splendid views out over County Donegal, to the beautiful gardens surrounding the Bishop's Gate Lodge. The lady responsible for these beautiful gardens was the warden, Jan Eccles. She was one of the most formidable and inspiring women that I had the great privilege to meet. Jan was an expert horticulturist with many qualifications and a lifetime's experience and expertise behind her. Jan was sixty years old when she arrived at Downhill and took up residency in the charming gate lodge (which survived a lot better than the castle, which is in ruins).

Unfortunately Jan suffered many break-ins and on one particular occasion when she thought she was being broken into, she waved her left arm in the air and thought she saw somebody but it was the fluorescent hands of her watch which was making the menacing shadows! She recounted this story to me with great glee. At a ripe old age Jan undertook a massive planting project, which thankfully she was able to see to fruition. When I arrived at Downhill, Jan was eighty nine years young and was still very much in charge. I have fond memories of her scaling trees to trim them, not trusting anyone else with the task. However it was clear that Jan was in need of some help, though she'd be the last to admit it. So I managed to gather a gang of volunteers together to get some of the larger jobs attended to. I got my crew from the university, and as I was studying

Geography and History, it was not hard to find willing participants. Under Jan's strict instructions and supervision we managed to clear a large area of mud and trim some of the larger trees. Jan rewarded us all at the end of it with tea and scones, which went down very well indeed!

Away from the charmed surroundings of Mussenden, I worked Portstewart Strand selling membership – it was basically cold selling conservation membership, sidling up to people as they were picnicking and giving them the nicest woman in the world routine. I tried to recruit Dolores into this job but she didn't last very long because of her alcoholism which made her sleep in most mornings. Also her style of recruiting new members was to wear a low cut top and flash her cleavage – all in all she was a total waste of space, but the beach was beautiful.

Seagulls

I can make the seagulls cry
By standing in the wind
For as they cry, they pass you by
Same breath with which we're twinned

Cry seagull you bird of shore
There's many more of you
I won't complain nor leave you lame
On this terrific view

The bird's the same
The coast it's plain
Will never better be
But our relationship has sunk
Off the rocks on Portstewart Sea

The Parting

calmly we said goodbye,
waiting till we passed,
but not our hearts.

and the sea rolls on,
and the waves ensure
that time also
carries on.

two gulls struggle against a breeze

but are parted
by forces that desire and human strength
cannot withstand.

and so we spoke the words,
leaving emotion for another time.

In my time at Portstewart Strand, there was a team of female recruiters. There was also a hideous male chauvinist pig. We were a separate entity from this character, but he seemed to think he could run rough shod over us as some kind of 'boss' figure. He, unsurprisingly, used to be a Sergeant Major in the army and his dictatorial nature came with him to Portstewart Strand. He was a major squealer, telling our boss in Belfast that I was hiding in the hut instead of parading around the beach on a scorching hot day (I had a very good medical reason for this. The antipsychotic drug that I was on – Largactil - produces extreme photosensitivity and sunburn; I was not ducking my duties). Another annoyance that came my way was scheduling my fortnightly depot injection of Depixol, and also the very fact that I was on any medication in the first place from my boss. Thankfully, he was not around every day, spending most of his time in Belfast. Despite the various oppositions and obstacles I encountered on my time cold calling on Portstewart Strand, I actually turned out to be the most successful recruiter! It must have been my irresistible charm and honesty that won me that accolade.

Carrick a Rede Rope Bridge was another tourist attraction I became familiar with – also cold calling the tourists. The organisation planted us there from St Patrick's Day onwards, and to say that the weather was a tad chilly would be an understatement! One time we had to give an exhibition of the charms of the North Coast in Coleraine Leisure Centre. Unfortunately some joker stole all of our huge posters of scenic pictures and the exhibition was a wash out because we had literally nothing to exhibit! On that long, boring and cold day I made friends with a man who was running a stand for Cancer Research. He was a lovely chap, but rather ironically he used to sneak out for a quick smoke with me whenever we had the chance. Brrrrrrrr! They were some chilly smokes!

At the Giant's Causeway it was a little bit claustrophobic because we were standing about in the centre all day with hundreds of tourists trekking in and out that were not recruitable because they were from a foreign country. On the upside, the Giant's Causeway had a beautiful craft centre and a wonderful cafe but they were, in my mind, a bit expensive. One lady who worked in the centre was from Ballycastle and talked about the 'staines' when she was referring to the Giant's Causeway stones. Nobody could understand her and it gave me a bit of a giggle in the cloistered surroundings of the centre. I regretted the fact that my foreign language skills would not pass muster as the centre at the Giant's Causeway was very cosmopolitan and I could have had some terrific conversations had I been able to speak any language other than English.

Chapter Six Friends and Lovers

In the meantime, whilst at home with my mother in 1979, I met somebody with whom I could have a relationship with, we shall use a code name to protect the innocent and call her Anne. Anne was a dark blonde or a dirty fair, not quite on the level of peroxide blonde in any case. She was terrifically funny and had an exceedingly humorous personality. We used to go out on adventures, usually to the pub, by bicycle. We never had a sexual relationship but we were close in every other way.

I had met Anne at Port Na Happle cafe in Portstewart. It was an absolutely beautiful place to eat lunch but it is now a residence at the very edge of the sea. I met her when I was a mere spring chicken of nineteen or twenty. This was a period of my life between universities; Anne was a year younger than me.

My mum's house was at the top of a hill and we used to cycle down to the pub which was located one mile away at the bottom of the hill. I challenged Anne to ride down to the pub without touching the pedals of the bicycle. She accomplished this and we managed to do it because there was a big dip in the hill. You couldn't do it nowadays because there is a big roundabout in the way. Anyway, when we got to the pub the fun was only beginning. We met up with two Bradford lads; well half Bradford, half Portstewart. The craic was mighty as we were sending up their swearing. The more they swore the more we swore back at them. After several pints we rode home on our trusty bicycles. We got as far as the police station in Portstewart and I was laughing so much I fell off the bicycle, quickly followed by Anne falling off hers too, in fits of laughter.

I visited Anne in England and passing through Belfast on the way home by train and boat I wrote 'A Rainy Day in Belfast'.

A Rainy Day in Belfast

A rainy day in Belfast
Still glistens in my mind,
The train pulls past the gasworks
As I think my friend is kind.

Our parting was so cheerful
A hug, a kiss, a smile.
We weren't even tearful,
Think I'll see her in a while.

The rain can batter all it wants
But will not wet us now,
Nor seek to wash away our faults
As the train pulls past another halt.

The water will only breathe new life
The sun will reappear,
And we shall settle all our strife
We shall not run from fear.

A rainy day in Belfast
Will glisten in my mind.

It was like daggers in my heart when her mother did not allow her to see me any more because she thought we were too close. But her mother held the purse strings so she really could not see me. I met Anne a few years ago, she'd recently remarried a widower with three young children, plus her boy from the first marriage. They were living out in the country, a somewhat secluded life. This seemed a strange fate to me for the outgoing, bubbly girl she had been.

Although perhaps not aware of it at the time, this was

my first lesbian love. However my next encounter with romance was not till after I got my degree from Coleraine University. I started a Masters Degree course in Peace and Human Conflict Studies at the Magee Campus in Derry. I also moved into a flat in Church Street, just behind the Promenade in Portstewart. I shared the flat with another girl, Dolores. We'd met at a friend's house. Dolores was from Belfast and had long blonde tumbling locks. I was immediately drawn to her. She had an air of easy sophistication that only city dwellers seem to have. Probably due to my obvious infatuation, she loved to poke fun at me with her sharp witty humour. Sharing the flat did not last as Dolores left to marry her boyfriend, a marriage which was annulled eight months later. Dolores returned to a flat in Church Street and we picked up where we had left off. The marriage had not ended amicably; Dolores was forced to get an exclusion order out against her former husband. One evening whilst at her flat he came to the door, and upon seeing me he flew into a wild rage. Through a mixture of fear and panic I pushed him with all the force I could muster, and he crashed to the bottom of the stairs.

In the silence that followed the blood drained from my

face as the reality of what I had done hit me; could I have killed him? A wave of relief flooded over me as I heard his groans coming from the bottom of the stairs. The things we do for love...

Being Wrong

In an island off an island
On the west coast of Europe
I find myself obsessed with you
Give me reasons apart from
my reasoning, for an answer
to all this.

Caught upon a wave of frustration
and anger I drove her husband
down the stairs. I punched
him and kicked him
You then punish me.

In an island off an island
On the west coast of Europe
I find myself regretting all the
energies and thought I spent on you.

All the reasons I had,
All the arguments I convinced
myself with
To end up nearly killing someone

How can I be so wrong?

However the relationship with Dolores was not all tears. I had met her in Jim's flat, Jim was a bit of a socialist and allowed anybody to stay in his flat whilst his girlfriend was in America. We had wild parties which involved illicit drugs, alcohol to fuel all night discussions where we put the world to rights. It was during one of these gatherings that Dolores and I met and forged what was to be a tumultuous relationship, but also a very important one.

Out of the Blue

It came out of the blue
Your soft lips beckoning me,
Pleading me to kiss.

And gradually out of the blue
I wanted to

I wanted to kiss.

Holding you there
You made me feel so worthy
So electric at the same time.
Carrying you up the stairs
I'd felt so strong,
But so concerned for you.
Then out of the blue
We kissed.

I still remember that kiss
You kept on saying as I trembled
That you loved me
"I love you, love you," you said.
My words could not form
But I wanted you,
I wanted you to kiss.

Later we tried to form our impressions,
To work out the connections
Of our love and our friendship
I told you not to worry
That I could not think of love-making with you.

Now I lie in bed, I think of you.

I feel myself soft, white, wet and warm.

So warm you would melt in it

So you could sleep on it,

So porcelain white you'd need dark glasses,

So wet you would drown in it.

I lie in bed

And inside I cry,

I missed you, I miss you.

I imagine how it would feel,

I think of your eyes

That can disturb me.

I want your eyes, your smiling eyes

To smile at me.

Our relationship had a very tentative start, we were on and off like a hot and cold tap as we each tried to find our way. Being in a lesbian relationship in a small town in Northern Ireland in the early nineties was very difficult. Homophobic bigotry was a unifying factor across the sectarian divide. Alcohol was often the only way to feel brave enough to show any kind of public affection. One evening in a bar in Coleraine, which was certainly not gay friendly, drunk and exuberant we ran outside   and kissed frantically in a doorway, like naughty schoolgirls. A car passing by several times only heightened the excitement of our illicit moment. However, we were first and foremost great friends, and more than anything we loved to have fun and laugh a lot.

I'll never forget when Dolores's much loved cat Kit died. Not the easiest cat to love – as she had quite a violent streak, and liked to scratch most visitors. Somehow I managed to get on her good side. When she died Dolores was very upset, more so than one would expect for a cat of her years. Early one morning I got a frantic call from Dolores telling me of the cat's demise and demanding that I take her to Glenkit to bury Kit! So off we headed under Dolores's directions first to Belfast, then out the Larne Road to Glenarm. We stopped at a Forest Park and Dolores ventured into the forest with a black bin bag containing Kit and a spade which she'd borrowed from my mother. Now this was in the middle of January, so after five hours of waiting, worrying and impending darkness, I had to phone the police. The police turned up and were preparing a search and rescue mission when Dolores came sauntering up. She was delighted with all this attention, and even I took great joy in getting to sit in the police car and seeing all the gadgets! Life with Dolores had never a dull moment!

For five years we continued with this charade of a romance, but looking back, I think I always knew Dolores' heart was not in the relationship. Through her darkest hours and bouts of homelessness, she would return to me, knowing I would always take her in and support her. I loved to treat Dolores to meals out and drinks, however she began to feel that this was my way of controlling her. The final nail in our relationship was an incident at a party. Dolores had had a lot to drink and was being very amorous. I knew she was too drunk for anything but passing out in bed. Having spent the night together with nothing happening, she convinced herself that I had taken advantage of her in a vulnerable state. Jim was at the party as well, and did all he could to inflame the situation by taunting Dolores over her relationship with me. The following morning I made Dolores an Ulster fry, our last supper, then drove her to her mother's. She finally found the strength to be honest and end the relationship. Even though it was over something that never happened, we both sadly knew it was the right decision.

It was eight years before I embarked on another lesbian relationship. I had become more active and involved in the lesbian scene in Belfast. I thought it would be a good way to meet someone special, and at least it provided me with a supportive and busy social life. Karaoke was my speciality; I would go to Belfast every Saturday to a very lively gay bar, a place like one would never find anywhere on the North Coast. I established a bit of a reputation as a gay karaoke singer and won lots of competitions. The prize was usually a bottle of vodka, which I don't drink. Unsurprisingly I always knew someone willing to snaffle it up! At a lesbian barbecue organised by a lesbian support group I met Kate, a divorced mother of four. Kate was certainly not a typical lesbian, she was what might be described as a lipstick dyke as she was very feminine, almost motherly. I guess with four children it came naturally to her, and I was very receptive to that part of her personality. There was an instant connection between us like an electric spark, she listened to me attentively all evening and seemed genuinely interested in my varied career. At the end of the evening I gave her my card, hoping that this would not be the last we would see of each other. When she phoned me that night, it gave me the first real glimmer of hope for a relationship.

What I Would Paint

What I would paint is a sea of green,
Where I've been before,
A sea of green, a sky of blue and a beach of golden
sand.

Then I lay on the sand and hold your hand,
And tell you that I'm true.

Until you decide what to do.

From that phone call my relationship with Kate
blossomed and involved a lot of to-ing and fro-ing
between Portstewart and Belfast. Kate and I spent a lot
of time walking on Benone Beach, an old haunt of
Kate's, windswept but invigorating, often taking a flask
of coffee and a sleeping bag to ward off the elements. I
will always remember that kiss under the sleeping bag
in the rain. The third person in this relationship was
Kate's West Highland terrier Dido! I got on very well
with the dog despite being a cat person, however, my
cat Bebe was not amused by this strange creature in

her territory who had the nerve to steal her food!

Kate and I lived in very different worlds. She had to two teenagers living at home and a difficult relationship with her ex husband. I know that her relationship with me and our time together were an escape, even a haven from the trials and tribulations of life. However this was Kate's relatively new foray into the world of lesbian relationships and she had not fully come to terms with this new part of her life. She increasingly tried to change me and was not happy with some of my lifestyle choices, namely drinking and smoking. Kate was a recovering alcoholic, so I did sympathise with this aspect of her drive to better me. But as a very light drinker, I really didn't feel the need to address my drinking. As for smoking, as far as I was concerned it was my only vice and I wasn't going to give it up.

Wanting

I remember when I used to wake you with a cup of tea,
Concerned you'd had a good sleep.
I gently opened the blue curtains,
And kissed you on the lips.

I would have cooked you breakfast,

Only you wanted cereal.

I never seemed to hit it right,

Never got you what you wanted, when you wanted it,

Never really knew what you wanted, at any particular time

But we did have each other

When times were bad,

We would have had each other.

Eventually we grew distant. Her visits to me became more infrequent and I began to resent forking out for a B&B when I went to see her. She would not allow me stay with her children in the house. Finally Kate admitted what we both knew; she didn't love me. To add insult to injury, she came out with this just before Valentine's Day!

I Feel

I feel foolish, devastated,

Not that I anticipated,

All my hopes negated,

Can't help feeling agitated.

You really should have waited,
Thought our feelings had been stated.

You and I not an item,
Pretending this is not happening
Didn't think we'd take a shattering,
Aspirations took a battering.

If you think it doesn't matter, Try for a new Valentine
And not the latter.

My relationship with Kate was my last romantic relationship. I have kept active in the Lesbian scene in Belfast, attending different events, and I am a regular at the Karoke at the gay bar in Belfast (a regular winner of this event too!) I also am in contact with various women through a lesbian forum, so I am certainly not lonely. And miraculously I did rekindle my friendship with Dolores after twelve years. The friendship lasted for eighteen months until one night, Dolores discovered that I knew her telephone number. I had mentally stored it since a phone call Dolores made in my presence to the

Housing Executive. In was in my memory for three months until my friend Mary was at my house and wanted to give Dolores a ring. I gave her the number, but we used caller withhold function. Unfortunately after the phone call Mary, who has a reputation for blabbing, told Dolores that I had access to her number.

On the Saturday night after Ash Wednesday, I rang Dolores with two rings on her land line to see if she was coming to visit me in my flat that evening. She rang back in an absolutely livid temper. I knew right then that it was all over. Her ferocity was so extreme I felt like harming myself, something that I had never really done before. I ran a bath, got a blade and phoned her back. Dolores did not believe I was in the bath so I splish splashed the water to let her know I wasn't joking. I actually had a razor blade in one hand while I was holding the phone in the other hand. I was intent on committing suicide which I saw as a natural extreme reaction to her extreme cruelty. The blade slipped out of my hand and fell down my behind my back so I couldn't get at it. Obviously this was going to be a botched suicide attempt! Then I realised I was still wearing my watch and it seemed important to get out of the bath to avoid damaging it. But then hey! I was killing myself any way so why bother? I hung up and tried to get the blade as deep as possible into my arms to reach the veins and arteries but alas, I lacked the courage to go through with it. Dolores was utterly oblivious to all of this.

On the Monday, I went to the front door of her house and showed her my arms. She came round to my flat on the Tuesday with Mary and proceeded to give me a good scolding. She said I needed a kick around the block. I knew in my heart this was the last time she would be here. A week after Ash Wednesday, I tried to leave her some heat pads for her bad back but she turned her nose up at them. It didn't stop there, this was one almighty lover's tiff! The next day we had a huge bust up. Dolores had the keys to my flat to feed my cat when I was away and she suddenly decided she wanted to return them to me. She kept me waiting like a lemon outside her flat and would not let me in. A key throwing match broke out between the two of us. She kept throwing the keys out of the window into the garden. I would pick them up and bring them up to her. Finally the keys were left in the garden. A fortunate soul mowing Dolores's lawn found them a few days later and put them on the bench inside the hall. Feeling rather recalcitrant, I bought Dolores a bunch of flowers and a card. In it I wrote 'Sorry, sorry, sorry, a thousand times sorry! You have my unreserved apologies'. She took the flowers in. 'Success!' I thought. But there was silence. I wanted to provoke a reaction from her so I put money through her letterbox. She went into melt down and screwed up a twenty pound note and threw it down the stairs in the hallway.

I still loved her no matter how mean she was to me. In another attempt at reconciliation, on Easter Sunday 2011 I put a chocolate golden Easter bunny on her door step and then I rang her to see if she had got it. While I was telling her that I loved her, and I always loved her and she was beautiful, attractive and intelligent and wonderful – basically extolling her every virtue, she told me to go away, commit suicide and this time make a better job of it. As if that wasn't enough, she told me to drop dead, move on because she had moved on and basically fuck off! So I took her at her word. On the Wednesday after Easter Sunday I rang Dolores and told her I was headed for the Bann shore to put stones in my pocket and walk into the river. As soon as I put my phone down, my mobile rang. Believe me, I had every good intention of walking into the Bann that night but miraculously my mobile phone suddenly rang and on it was a friend from Belfast who managed to convince me to stay in this mortal coil a while longer. The best advice she gave me was to go to the pub and forget about Dolores – the age old remedy for a broken heart. When I was three quarters down the way of my shandy the Police suddenly appeared on the scene looking for me. There but for the grace of God I was not sectioned!

Chapter Seven Masters

In 1992 I finally graduated with honours from the University of Ulster at Coleraine. I was elated to have achieved this feat after all the rather exhaustive trials and tribulations I had endured over the previous years trying to get a degree. This achievement gave me the courage and the ambition to go on to do a Masters Degree at the University of Ulster Magee Campus in Derry in Peace and Human Conflict Studies. My MA dissertation looked at the rate of Psychiatric morbidity during the Northern Ireland Conflict. I discovered that as the homicide rate goes up the suicide rate goes down and inversely so.

During my Masters I took up a position with The National Schizophrenia Fellowship. My job title was Voices Development Officer. This role entailed establishing support groups throughout the Western Health and Social Services Board. I absolutely loved the job as it involved so much variety and diversity. It entailed a lot of travelling but I met great people and I really felt that I was contributing and making a positive difference to survivors' lives.

However, prejudice never fails to follow the so called 'different' person wherever they go – and even here in my role as a campaigner for the underdog my sexuality was seen as a threat and I learnt that to be openly gay in the workplace was an impossibility. During a meeting with my boss I was asked to recite some of my poetry. I recited a poem called 'Waiting in the Lobby', which gives an insight into the psychiatric system from the survivor's perspective. Then to offset the sombre and harrowing subject matter of that poem, I recited a beautiful love poem 'Out of the Blue' written about a first lesbian kiss. However it was this poem that proved to be my downfall. As soon as I had finished I realised that all was not well; she asked me if the person I referred to in the poem was female. Foolishly I said yes, I hadn't time to cover my tracks and perhaps I didn't fully comprehend that her manner and tone screamed out homophobia and disapproval. This was followed by a visit out of the blue to my home, however this time when my boss questioned me I was ready. She asked me 'if I had any physical liaisons with women'. Like the notorious womaniser Bill Clinton, I bluntly said no!

During my Masters I decided to move to Derry, hoping to immerse myself in student life and what I believed to be a good social scene. Tragically at this time there was very little going on in Derry, due mainly to the Troubles and the heavy presence of the British army on the streets and even around the campus. One felt constantly watched, observed and ill at ease. I found myself also being taunted about my religion by another student in the student bar, which was quite Republican at the time. This further added to my unease and paranoia. Another incident around that time further illustrated the danger of this city. A French bluegrass band came and played in the university's student's union and brought some much needed fun. I danced all night and felt all my worries ease in that magical way that music seems to do to a person. I was sickened to the pit of my stomach when I found out the next day that their van and all their equipment had been burnt out. Around this time there was the Halloween Trick or Treat massacre in Greysteel in County L'Derry. I went to the peace rally afterwards in the Derry air and I wrote this poem about the rally which was subsequently published in the Derry Journal:

The Peace Rally:

The rain came down,

There's a rally in the town,

Tears of Greysteel shed,

In the City in the wet,

Names of dead read out,

As we gathered about,

Words of Peace spoke,

While we got soaked.

But warmth was there,

In the Derry air (Guildhall Square)

We all shook hands,

For peace in our land,

Solidarity in grief

With the bereft,

The rain had stopped,

By the time we left.

As I remembered,

Silence is peace,

Peace in the square.

During this time my mother's health deteriorated. She was suffering from Transient Ischemic attacks and I was forced to move closer to home to help care for her. So I returned to Portstewart, my old stomping ground. It was then that I moved in to a flat in Church Street with Dolores. Shortly after Dolores moved out and I lived on my own in Church Street for the next five years. During this time I was always on call to my late mother, as our roles were sadly reversed and I became the one to care and worry for her. The rest of my family were busy with their jobs, their children and their responsibilities. Two of them now lived abroad, and another one in Belfast. So despite my history of illness I now had to shoulder this responsibility alone and make sure my mother received the care she needed. My mother needed me to drive her to various appointments as she was now confined to a wheelchair. My role as a carer became full time, so it was a mighty struggle to keep on top of my Masters, whilst also working for the NSF. It is only with hindsight that I realise all that I miraculously managed to do during this time – all the balls I managed to juggle without dropping one, but perhaps my Masters and work were necessary diversions for me at the time and gave me the strength to achieve my goals. All I can attest to is watching a parent decline and waste away before your eyes is one of the most difficult experiences any of us will go through.

When I submitted my Masters dissertation I was on my way to Galway for a brief sojourn with a friend. One of her friends thought I appeared psychotic on the trip because I was falling asleep over my pint! I didn't understand this logic but when I came back from Galway I really did start losing the plot. I believe that this was a reaction to all the stress and strain I had been under during the past year. My psychosis manifested itself as staying up all night and having no sleep. I had zilch functioning the next day, clinging to my coffee cup and chain smoking like a chimney. My responsibilities were too great and I had a post dissertation crisis. I had managed to hold everything together in order to hand in my dissertation. Once I had achieved that everything came crashing down, and I was once again in the abyss. Sleep eluded me as I became more and more manic, and I would spend the night smoking frantically. When I ran out of cigarettes I became desperate. In the morning I would knock or should I say bang on my neighbours' door to ask for some cigarettes, It was clear to them that I was in a very bad way. I was aware that I needed help and I knew that I would have to be admitted to a psychiatric ward before I lost all control. When I phoned my CPN she advised me that I could only be admitted if I was suicidal. I promptly informed her that if I was not admitted to hospital, I would jump off Coleraine Bridge, and that was no idle threat. I was taken seriously and my GP had me admitted by ambulance to the local psychiatric unit. My stay there lasted four dreary months.

Once there I was heavily medicated as is the norm for most patients who enter the unit. The drugs I was given led to weight gain (surprise surprise!), however I managed to stick to a strict diet and I kept a good portion of the weight off. Times were not all grim; I managed to make some good friends. A woman also called Carole was in the bed next to me. We got on like a house on fire and behaved like young teenagers. We giggled so much together that we were seen by the staff as a bad influence on each other. They thought that we brought out each other's mania. But I believe laughter is also great therapy, much needed in a place as dour as a psychiatric unit, and to have friendships with people who understood this illness was very empowering for both of us.

Although I had completed my dissertation, in order to graduate it had to be bound and three copies submitted. Although still not very well I was desperate to graduate, after all the trials and tribulations I had suffered to get there. From the hospital I had the difficult task of trying to organise for a university secretary to do this for me. As this was in the days before mobiles, I had to use the hospital phone to make these arrangements. Wouldn't you believe it! A particularly nasty nurse tried to sabotage my efforts, doing particularly mean things like cutting off my calls at every opportunity. His sadistic streak also included blocking off the lounge area to patients at night, a very cruel trick as so many of us did not sleep well, and a cigarette during these long dark nights of the soul was our only comfort. After much capering and antics, I was successful in getting my dissertation bound and submitted and was also granted permission to leave the hospital for the day to attend my graduation from Magee College, Derry.

Leaving a psychiatric ward to attend one's graduation ceremony may not sound ideal, but both the staff and patients managed to make it a very special and memorable day. The nurses (not including the nasty one!) made a real fuss of me, they did my hair and make up and made sure that I looked a million dollars for my big day. As I was leaving the patients lined up and formed a guard of honour and gave me an enormous round of applause, some were even crying! Both my mum and brother attended the ceremony with me at the Guildhall in Derry. I was delighted that my mother could attend as she was quite frail at this time and in a wheelchair. However, my brother decided to go off to see the city walls, leaving me minding my mum and missing out on the strawberries and cream! A vital rite of passage at every graduation day! But it was a proud day as I was one of only a handful from my class who had managed to achieve the Masters Degree.

We had a celebratory meal afterwards where alcohol was banned! However, I then had to return to the hateful hospital and do battle with my demons once more. I was to languish in hospital for a further four weeks. But I was not going to let a little thing like hospitalisation beat me. My next grand project was to try to organise my attendance at the World Congress for Mental Health which was being held at Trinity College, Dublin that year. Yet again I faced an onslaught of opposition and abuse from the world's nastiest psychiatric nurse (I was beginning to feel like a super hero trying to do battle with him!) while I was attempting to use the hospital phone to arrange accommodation and liaise with the National Schizophrenia Fellowship who were sponsoring me to attend. Although they agreed to sponsor me they also asked for my resignation, as unfortunately their funding had been cut. So whilst delighted at the prospect of attending this event, it was a bittersweet victory.

I had only been released from hospital two weeks when I was thrust into the daunting task of travelling to Dublin and negotiating this busy city on my own. I stayed in a hostel and spent each day at the more luxurious surroundings of Trinity College. The organisers underestimated the numbers attending the survivor led part of the conference where I was speaking, and a couple of hundred people where herded into a very small room. This was distressing for people who would find such an event difficult in itself, without the added pressure of being in such a confined space. However, when I stood to speak I found my nerve and recited my poem 'Waiting in the Lobby'. This poem describes my experiences of being in a psychiatric hospital and gives an insight into my fears and emotions and how I felt coming out the other side.

Reciting this poem earned me a standing ovation. It also signified the end of a journey for me, a validation of all my experiences. I had a come out the other end with a better understanding of my illness, and of myself. My poetry had played a huge part in this. Poetry was a very cathartic and healing process, and it became my life's work to promote this amongst other survivors.

Carol E Kelly

Chapter Eight Dissertation Days

During my MA/PgDip in Peace and Human Conflict I worked as Voices Development Officer for the National Schizophrenia Fellowship (NSF) for the Strabane and Derry area. As part of my job, I formed support groups for the mentally ill – all over the Western Health Board – from Limavady to Enniskillen. I once took Dolores to a meeting. We had been shopping in Belfast and we were to go to Omagh but I mistakenly took the wrong motorway. We ended up having to backtrack and I, for the first time in my life, experienced a bout of road rage. Dolores then got road rage at my road rage and I had to settle down. We arrived 25 minutes late to a meeting in Omagh. Dolores thought that she could hide in the kitchen, but oh no, I made her participate in the meeting!

I had great success with my advocacy and support group work, I loved my job and I was good at it. Unfortunately, due to lack of funds, the job was made obsolete and that was the end of my time with the National Schizophrenia Fellowship. The only negative thing that happened during my work with the NSF was a stupid decision I made to contravene the rules and take home one of the members of a support group who tried to rape me. The problem was that in my job, I became very friendly with the people in support groups and perhaps over-empathised with them too much, being a psychiatric patient. That was the only stain on my time with the NSF.

When I was doing my MA dissertation, I was living in 11 Church Street, otherwise known as Amytiville because it was a non stop living psychodrama being played out in Portstewart. In this heady atmosphere, my dissertation began to take shape when I found out about some interesting social concepts. These included merited fate, which means that if someone gets shot in the street, he somehow deserved it – in other words you deserve what you get and you get what you deserve. Then there is denial throughout society and government, and each paramilitary organisation denied humans of their lives too. The ordinary people denied that times were so hard and that they were so bereft. Denial can also be denial of one's responsibilities, for example, through alcohol or suicide.

I came up with the Seven Theories:

1) People assume that they cannot be helped by the mental health system, i.e. it won't bring back

loved ones killed in the violence – so they don't enter hospital. There is no point in reporting to the authorities as it cannot bring a loved one back.

2) Emigration – a lot of people emigrated to escape the Troubles.

3) Habituation – the people of Northern Ireland basically became accustomed to violence – to bombs and gunshots.

4) Latency period – here there is a delayed reaction in which a person feels the emotions quite some time after the harrowing event has taken place. This is like an after shock when the burden of coping is lifted.

5) External stress rather than internal stress. Street rioting in the early 1970s was external aggression, so therefore internal aggression decreased and the number of those who presented themselves to psychiatrists lessened.

6) Cohesion in the community against outsiders – the idea of being watched and observed by the army was rife in the Troubles in both communities, engendering a paranoia against

perceived outsiders who may be part of the 'enemy'.

7) As the homicide rates increased, the suicide rates decreased and inversely so. With peace we have more suicides.

Meanwhile, back at 11 Church Street, my head was all over the place. Dolores was coming on to me and also marrying her boyfriend whom she had known for a mere three months. The marriage lasted five months and was slowly annulled. During her wedding day, the bride and groom were both intoxicated on brandy. They went to a dive bar for the reception where Dolores proceeded to throw her wedding ring at him. I was not invited to the wedding, and they had difficulty finding witnesses at the last minute. Throughout her nuptial adventures, Dolores did not speak to me but I came to her rescue whenever she was left homeless and high and dry after the marriage broke up. I took her in and fed her, even giving up my bed for her. The nefarious groom Alex broke into the back of my flat where the bedrooms were and stole Dolores's duvet and clothes. He threw them in the dustbin outside. Dolores had a taste for Tequila and I was always willing to satisfy her needs. I would buy her double and triple Tequilas at the bar. She threw them into her pint and other people's pints too! She cried when the duvet and pillow were thrown into the dustbin because they had to be washed and did not smell of Alex any more. We had to wait up with our shoes on in the living room until this mess with Alex blew over. Dolores's cat was finely tuned into what a bastard Alex was; she would hiss, spit and even growl when he turned up at the door.

Dolores and I liked to frequently travel around the Antrim coast. Our favourite haunt was Kenbane Castle. We took a picnic there and plenty of photographs. Dolores, although very photogenic, was extremely hard to take photographs of because she hated having her photo taken, but we managed to take some terrific snaps of her at Kenbane Castle. Alex would later steal them.

The people who are closest to you are often the last to know or pick up on things about loved ones. I had no clue that Dolores was a slave to the demon drink. I didn't notice either that she was anorexic because often drunks do not eat. So I felt really good treating her to meals. There was one restaurant in Portrush that offered a dessert she loved – Baked Alaska - and it made me so happy to see her eat as she weighed a meagre six and a half stones. Dolores was brave and fond of any and every drink, but even she, at this stage of her life, was getting sick of alcohol and frustrated that she couldn't live without it. When she was out in the pub, she would throw drinks around her in disgust when she was inebriated – usually into other people's pints! She showed signs of self hatred and let old men feel her breasts. On alcohol Dolores would get very amorous. On one drunken occasion she went to bed with the old socialist Jim and a female Spanish friend. Our Dolores loved a threesome. At one stage, she begged me to go to bed with her and Alex. On the occasion when she went to bed with Jim and his Spanish senorita, Elvis walked in, a man who is two sandwiches short of a picnic, and began crying at his lack of participation in the ménage a trois.

After my dissertation was finished, I went to stay with a friend in Buncrana, County Donegal who was in the process of leaving her husband. I knew her husband very well and we ended up having an affair. The husband was also mentally ill. We took no precautions and after four weeks, I realised that I was pregnant – in fact I had conceived on Friday 13th October – a most inauspicious date.

Whenever I got back To Portstewart, I contacted my GP and psychiatrists. I was admitted to a psychiatric clinic and after eight weeks, I was shown a photographic scan of the foetus. I was advised by the doctors that the baby was would have been severely deformed had it gone to full term, hence a termination was necessary. Upon seeing the pictures and hearing this devastating news, I remarked to the gynaecologists 'It's life Jim but not as we know it'. I guess that this rather morbid humour was my way of dealing with the situation. Ultimately, the termination was the best decision for both the foetus and myself, particularly as the baby would have had no decent father figure. After the termination, I was to rescue the father from homelessness in Derry. He came to live in Portstewart but things between us were very acrimonious. He ventured back to Derry pretty swiftly and I haven't seen hide nor hair of him since.

Whenever I had finished my MA in Peace and Human Conflict Studies at Magee, I had a burning desire to do a PhD in the field of psychiatric nursing from the patient's perspective. In order to do this I had to take final year nursing research modules at the University of Ulster at Coleraine. I managed to scrape through these modules and I started a PhD by publication with Professor Mary Chambers, who was an expert in psychiatric nursing. Unfortunately, she didn't have enough time for me and she was promoted to a higher standing in an English University. Down the drain went my PhD dreams.

During this time, I thought I would try my hand at lecturing. I sent my CV to the Psychology Department at Coleraine campus, Occupational Therapy at Jordanstown and Psychiatric Nursing at Magee. I was later to get a part time temporary contract with the social work department at Magee. I tried the medical school at Queen's University, Belfast but they put up barriers. My lecturing work at Magee and the social work department involves giving presentations on the fears and the needs of the psychiatric patient, and also lecturing on the stigma and discrimination surrounding the mental patient. I like to involve my poetry in my lecturing and it always goes down a great storm!

Chapter Nine My TRAVELS

In 1999 and the year 2000 I began another academic adventure - studying modules in Nursing Research in order to do a doctorate in nursing from the patient's perspective. I scraped by in the Nursing Research modules because my head was all over the show. My mother had just passed away and I had various mental health issues bubbling away in the background. Nevertheless, I am blessed with the gift of the gab and I talked my way into starting a PhD by publication in nursing. My professor asked me to do a piece of work for a book in Psychiatric nursing which was eventually published. She also asked me to entertain some Canadian visitors who were psychiatric survivors from OCAB, the Ontario Council of Alternative Businesses. OCAB form businesses run for and by psychiatric survivors such a courier system throughout Toronto and cafes all over Ontario, as well as catering services.

When the four Canadian ladies from OCAB arrived at Coleraine it was my job to show them the scenic North Coast. Unfortunately I could not show them the Giants Causeway as being true city girls they were wearing very high unsuitable heels for the walks and the terrain of the Giants Causeway was not made for stiletto shoes! Two of the women were lesbians and one of them, Liz, took a real shine to me even though she had a partner sequestered away in Canada. We ended up enacting a Romeo and Juliet scene in the hotel she was staying at. Liz was up on the balcony shouting words of love to me and I was blowing her kisses. Such a tender moment!

I was so inspired by the women from OCAB's visit that I went to a regional newspaper and appealed for donations to visit OCAB in Canada for the purpose of studying how the businesses run by mentally ill people worked. Tom Beare MBE sponsored me to the tune of £3,000 to go to Toronto and realise my hopes and dreams. So in June 2002 I boarded a plane for Canada, and this is where I got the inspiration after September 11th 2001 for my poem Rush To Wait, which deals with the vexations of travelling after the said tragedy:

Rush to Wait

Rushing out at 3.30am
I realise this was all a joke
Rushing to the airport
To wait three hours for a Transatlantic flight

Rush to the airport

Wait on a seven and a half hour flight

Wait for the pilot

Wait for the refreshments

Rush to wait

Bad for the blood pressure

Then finally take off

My neighbouring passenger's

Rosary beads are keeping us up

At 60,000 feet

My nerves are frazzled from not smoking

I was too busy to sleep

Can't even doze

Because of the noise

The lady with the rosary beads

Has the right idea

She's got ear plugs

And now in Toronto city

I find it full of witty queers

Talking about their 'friends'

All this rushing to wait.

When I landed in Toronto I was a bag of nerves. Liz and her partner invited me out for a meal. I was so excited to go it amplified my lithium tremor considerably, just as if I had stuck my finger in a live electric socket. Thankfully I kept my cool and enjoyed a really juicy steak and a pint of Toronto lager – truly authentic Canadian cuisine! Unfortunately this proved to be the height of my entertainment at the hands of my Canadian hosts. I was just expected to go to work and then amuse myself in the evenings. Albeit, they did give me a mobile phone – but that was the height of it.

My first day's work was alongside Richard Costello, searching for little scurry, furry things like mice and rats. A little known fact – rats and mice detest tin foil – and this is what Richard and I used to discourage them from entering the premises. That was pretty good fun. Alas, the good times did not last forever. I was assigned to toilet cleaning duties. The toilets in Toronto had a certain smell of bleach which really got up my nose and lingered there. In the Centre for Addiction and Mental Health (CAMH), where OCAB have a cafe, called Out of This World, the toilets happened to be the world's vilest, most disgusting abominations that I have ever encountered in the lavatorial world. But I was fly; I sneaked up to the Executive suite and performed my ablutions in a rather more sanitary environment.

The first time I went to CAMH Centre for Addiction and Mental Health, I was not informed that it was a psychiatric hospital, but rather just a building. We got to ride in a cab with the sandwiches and coffee to a boardroom which was full of my favourite people – psychiatrists! On a later trip to CAMH we took a coffee cart around the forensic wards where the most dangerously ill patients were held in lock up wards. CAMH was a very important facility for me as it provided plenty of patients for me to interview for my PhD. For my study tour in Toronto, I was mainly based in The Raging Spoon which was a cafe run by psychiatric survivors.

Cast adrift in a big city I was very lonely, but at the same time I was determined to sample the delights of city life, chaperones or no chaperones. I ventured out to Church Street in Toronto, which is the premier gay area. I met a gay man who was seeking gay friendships from Belfast. What a small world! He took me to an exclusively male club. We walked in via a back entrance and I managed to get totally lost and exit out the front which was on a totally different street. I was baffled as to where I was and I asked somebody the way back to Church Street. Unfortunately, this gentleman turned out to be a queer-basher and he stalked me several streets until I nearly got back to my hotel. Within spitting distance of the hotel, this man asked me for money. When I declined his request he bashed me in the back. Fortunately, he did not have a knife. I collapsed to the ground, believing my teeth had been knocked out. I ended up with bruises on my knees and a very sore back and sore knees. Terrified he may do me further harm, I lay on the ground until my assailant went away. When I was sure he had vanished, I stumbled onto my feet and limped my way back to the hotel. At the hotel, I told the Night Porter what had happened. He asked me did I want to phone the police, but I declined. I was much too physically, mentally and emotionally battered and exhausted to deal with any further drama that night.

Waking up the next morning, I was relieved to discover that my attacker had not made off with any of my money which was in the region of $800. I had to inform my workplace of my injuries and of the attack. The secretary of OCAB, Pat, came out to see me as did the police. I was interviewed by the police and I managed to give them an extraordinarily detailed report of my attacker but alas, it was too late to catch him. If I had phoned the police the night before, there would have been a good chance that they could have picked him up as I was able to describe him to a T, including the colour of his eyes and the fact he was six feet four inches tall. Unfortunately the police had to drop it as the assailant would have disappeared in the vast city of Toronto.

My hotel was called Town in Suites. Nearby there was a pub I favoured called Spirits. It was there that I made a lot of friends. As Canadians were pioneers of the No Smoking in public places rule, we did all our smoking at Spirits outside. When it was raining, we huddled under the parasols. It was there I met my good friend Stacey, who upon hearing I had been mugged, promised me that she would organise for a group of us to go out to a gay night club on Saturday night and that I would be fully protected and safe. At the back of this nightclub there were pool tables and also an astonishing Ice Hockey table in which the puck would whizz by at such a speed you were in danger of breaking your fingers! One of my comrades that evening was a lesbian cop named Vicky. I told her I worked for OCAB and she wanted to know what the acronym stood for and she was curious as to what 'alternative' meant. I was a bit flabbergasted and did not know what to say as I did not want to mention the dreaded words 'mental health'. My minders went out of their way to see me off back to my hotel. That was a very jolly jaunt.

There was another drinking emporium called Slack Alice's. One time I went in to order a meal. As I spoke, a voice piped up "You're Irish! I'm Irish too!" (in a Canadian accent!). Her name was Susan Rose and she was from Newfoundland. We gabbled away the entire afternoon and then she came back to my hotel room. I told her that I had recently been mugged and my back was very sore. Susan offered me a back massage. An offer I could not resist! As a lusty woman, I blew my chances by coming on too strong for Susan's tastes. She fled in a hurry but I had her contact number. After she left me in the lurch, I decided a swim in the hotel's pool would cool my ardour and we arranged to meet up later. I found out that night that Susan had only got over the break up of a recent relationship and that is why she had bolted from my hotel room. Later on in the trip to Canada, I was invited over to Susan's place and I met her huge pedigree dog called Scotty. I didn't have a clue what sort of breed he was, but my god he was a muscular mountain! On my second trip to Canada, I was to share a bed with Scotty while I stayed with Susan, but with my illness she could not tolerate me being sick, so I had to go back to the hotel. On one particularly memorable evening I was sick and the dog ate it up! I thought that dogs only returned to their own vomit but Scotty was an exception to the rule!

CAMH possessed its own acting theatre on which I got the pleasure to perform my poetry – a poem entitled A Rainy Day in Belfast. They also discovered that I could sing! We all sang Crocodile Rock by Elton John, but I was the only one who knew the words. They singled me out for praise for my vocal talents! At Spirits, there was karaoke, and I gleefully got up on stage to perform Crocodile Rock again and Sinatra's My Way to a cheering audience. Later I would go back to Canada and take workshops in performance poetry so this was a sign of things to come.

I had the 'privilege' of working at OCAB's courier service – AWAY Express which was run by a manager who seemed to take a dislike to me. I had met a reporter from a major national Canadian news network who had expressed an interest in doing a story about me and my MA dissertation. She said that she would get back to me through the manageress of AWAY Express (who was our point of contact) but I never heard anything from her again. I believe it was a deliberate attempt by the manageress to sabotage my work in mental health advocacy. I should mention that this woman was highly unpopular among her staff.

My first trip to Canada was very informative and I had a party on the last day – lesbians only! I cooked an Irish stew but it didn't go down too well (literally) as Canadians don't like lamb. I had asked one of my lesbian friends to come to the party with a knife to cut up the lamb – they were on bicycles and had they been stopped by the police they would have been arrested for carrying a dangerous weapon! I returned the knife to Liz and we had a good old time of it.

Visit number two to Canada came about in March 2003 when the ADF (Arts and Disability Forum) sponsored me to go the Madness and Arts Festival 2003. At the festival I held a workshop with Pascale Reboul who is a French Canadian poet. She gave me her poetry book which is in French and entitled TerresD'Exil. The workshop was a fabulous success. I only had a short time to read and act out my poetry but it went down to great applause. I encouraged people in the audience who had poems of their own to act them out themselves but if they had stage fright, I enacted them out for them and this went down a treat. This was March and it should have been the Canadian winter time but it was unseasonably mild. The only memory that really stands out is walking up Church Street to say goodbye to Susan Rose in Spirits bar. And after I said goodbye, predictably as can be, the weather changed back to Arctic conditions.

My love affair with Canada was to continue for a third time. I took my friend Libby with me under the auspices of an Arts Council Award that I got to undertake poetry workshops in Canada. I introduced the first workshop with my performance poetry, and Libby gave some suggestions as to what everyone in the group could write about – through pictures in magazines. Sadly, on the third day of our stay in Canada, Libby announced her imminent departure for Ireland. She missed her boyfriend too much and basically took all of his money to get her home. What a disappointment. But still, I soldiered on, being the resilient character that I am, and took the second workshop on my own at which one of my students burst into song after reading her poem!

I should say at this point that during all of my visits to Canada I had visited my uncle, aunt and cousins who lived in Peterborough, Ontario. The final trip was undoubtedly the best because it was the fall. We sauntered round my uncle's farm and saw the beautiful leaves on the trees falling in the autumn sunshine. I am still in touch with my uncle and many of my Canadian friends. I owe a huge debt to Canada for teaching me so much.

After my Canadian adventures, I was soon to find myself in another far flung place on the globe. In 2006, I won an Arts Council Award to be Artist in Residence at a Nutter's Conference in Napier, North Island, New Zealand. I took with me Eileen Pollock, better known as Lilo Lil in Bread and the Money Lender in Angela's Ashes. Eileen has a house in Portstewart and we met in the Anchor Bar. I was unsuccessfully helping her with a crossword at the time. We jetted off to New Zealand, via Homeland Security in Los Angeles. The security sure was sensitive in LA as I'm sure you can imagine! So that was a twelve and a half hour flight followed by ANOTHER twelve and a half hour flight. My backside was getting rather numb.

We arrived in Auckland where we were greeted by Eileen's cousin. Before the conference, we had a few days' rest and I made the discovery that New Zealand has all black beaches and all black swans. We stayed in a B&B in Napier where the South Korean landlady rather unsuccessfully tried to convert me to Christianity. Finally, the conference rolled around. First of all, Eileen interviewed me in front of an audience about my life, my illness and my work. Afterwards I performed some of my poems. During the recital, I made a cheeky quip "Are there any Lesbians here?". The roar of approval that followed nearly lifted the ceiling! I read 'Out of the Blue', 'Waiting in the Lobby' and 'Ode to Cissy' amongst others. All in all, the first day of the conference was a brilliant success. My luck continued into the evening, when at the bar I met a Maori Lady named Joyce Renata. We talked and philosophised into the wee small hours of the night and Joyce announced to me and Eileen that I was her soul mate. False words they proved to be, for disaster struck when she met her soon to be long term Maori girlfriend the very next day! They were both mental health survivors.

Outside at the conference, there was a visual artist. You could paint whatever tickled your fancy. I painted a volcano as there were plenty of them in New Zealand. On the very last day of the conference, we had the great privilege to meet the Governor General of New Zealand.

We generally conversed about being nutters – he considered himself to be a nutter too! Outside on that last day, I was having a cigarette, minding my own business, when out of nowhere I was yanked by Joyce into the conference hall to recite a long poem without my book. I managed to do this successfully without crapping myself, although I had rivers of sweat trickling down my brow. After that piece of drama, I met the head of the New Zealand Mental Health Commission (who is also a survivor) and she gave me the times and venues for four poetry recitals in Wellington. Brimming with excitement and anticipation, Eileen and I boarded a bus with Alan Tucker, an Australian survivor – predictably there was a shortage of smoking and toilet facilities. We arrived during the working week and headed for a lesbian bar (where else would one head to?). By the Sunday I had managed to bag a gig at the lesbian bar too! Whilst I was in Wellington, Eileen and I stayed in an all women's hostel where we linked up with the landladies – a mother and daughter with her partner. The craic was mighty. Unfortunately I cannot recount much about the poetry recitals as they flashed by in a blur.

My time in Wellington had come to an end. It had been

a marvellous city. Never again would I ever taste a rack of lamb so mouth watering in any restaurant, but for those in Wellington! And never had so much champagne been drunk by Eileen (champagne was very cheap in New Zealand - Champagne Lil!) We had to return to Auckland where we once again met Eileen's cousin. It was time to fly home and face the gruelling, buttock-numbing twelve and a half hour flight to Los Angeles Homeland Security where we would be made to feel like a pair of America's Most Wanted. Then, we managed to avoid being pegged as couple of suicide bombers, and we had to go through the twelve and a half hour flight back home to Heathrow where we would kiss the ground after making it through such a torturous long haul journey.

Chapter Ten Media Activist

My initial media focus was based mainly around my sporting feats. It started back in 1975 in the Coleraine Chronicle which documented my numerous sporting successes. These included the Second Elevens Derry and Antrim championship for hockey and later in 1977, Ulster Senior School Girl Champion for discus and shot-putt. In 1981, I was in the papers again as I had been selected to play Volleyball for Northern Ireland. Then in 1980, I was featured on the front page of the Irish Times along with my rugby team as we were victorious in drubbing Trinity College rugby team on College Park. Perhaps my proudest sporting media moment came in the Coleraine Chronicle in 1980 where I was specially profiled as an athlete and for my sporting prowess. The article mentioned that I excelled not just in one sport, but in multiple sports including the Women's Volley Ball team at Jordanstown which helped organise the Northern Ireland League. Sadly some of the tournaments were thwarted due to the conflict in Dublin. I was awarded my international cap without having to play, as were the rest of the team. The article also chronicled my legendary win over Trinity College Dublin with the Rugby Team on College Park – 22 points to nil!

At that time I was preparing for the Northern Ireland 3As Championship, and that was detailed in the Chronicle article too. This also incorporated more sports – discus and shot-putt. The article even went on to mention my artistic talents and my love for writing poetry! I was exceedingly proud of this profile of myself. I was such a golden girl, my girlfriend at the time used to slag me rotten over it.

My career as a Mental Health journalist began in earnest in October 1994 in a Mental Health Magazine called Choice which was produced by the Western Area Health Board. At the time, I was working as a Development Officer for the National Schizophrenia Fellowship in that area. I told the magazine of my experiences as a mental health survivor, how difficult it was for me to strive for a university education in the face of my illness and I urged for the psychiatric establishment to listen to the voices of sufferers of mental illness. I espoused the idea of mental health sufferers meeting up in groups, an idea that I still hold close to my heart today. Finally, I spoke of the recuperative powers of music and poetry, another subject dear to me.

In April 1995, I appeared in the Derry Journal in an attempt to change public attitudes about schizophrenia. The article mentions my achievements – sporting, academic and artistic, which is in contrast to the stereotypical average public view of schizophrenics and what they can achieve with their lives. The article stresses that it was not all plain sailing for me, I had to fight stigma and discrimination as well as coping with severe mental illness. However, I wanted to give a message of hope and reform the stereotypes of schizophrenia. This article was also written when I was a Development Officer with the National Schizophrenia Fellowship.

I was to appear in the Derry Journal one more time whenever I graduated with my MA from The University of Ulster Magee Campus.

Throughout the late 1990s and early 2000s I wrote many articles for Fortnight magazine which is a Belfast-based Northern Irish current affairs magazine. In July 1995, I wrote an article named 'Denial' – a major theme in my MA dissertation – about denial in government and society and the Troubles and what impact this would have for the people of Northern Ireland and their mental health. This article was based on a conference I attended called Conflict and Mental Health at Queen's University, Belfast. It was expected by Dr Peter Curran that more people would present with mental health problems due to the then recent ceasefire. I came to the conclusion that the mental health services had better steel themselves for an onslaught of patients presenting themselves to psychiatrists.

In October 1995 I had the pleasure to attend and subsequently to write about a highly controversial conference that was taking place at Trinity College, Dublin, in the Republic of Ireland – the World Federation for Mental Health. One of the delegates, in fact the keynote speaker - Professor Anthony Clare - gave a very illuminating talk on how the partnership between patients and doctors had been full of knavery and abuse equalled only by being the stigma of being a psychiatric patient. Ex patients faced discrimination from all sides in life. He said that compassion, patience, warmth and intelligence were the key ingredients to dealing with psychiatric patients. Dr John Alderdice, then the leader of the Alliance Party and also a psychiatrist, said that the cessation of conflict in Northern Ireland would bring enhanced psychiatric morbidity as it would cause internal warfare. At this conference, I read my signature poem, Waiting in the Lobby, and I got a standing ovation!

In September 1999, I wrote another piece for Fortnight magazine detailing the difficulties that the mentally ill have with co-habitation and marriage. 79.4% of psychotic patients remain unmarried, but there is a dearth of information as to why this is the case in Northern Ireland. Could it be that so many psychotic patients spend time in hospital during the years in which their 'normal' peers are founding relationships? What about the effect of psychiatric medication on female fertility, childbearing and the health of the foetus? Like any disability, a mental health problem can make or break a marriage. Hoofer (1986) suggests that the marriage may become stronger after a psychotic episode, but there is a paucity of research. Mentally ill people are supposed to have the same rights to work but they do not have the same rights in the divorce court as a mother or father. In Northern Ireland, this crucial area has not been explored and further evidence is required for a conclusion.

In February 2001, I wrote in Fortnight magazine about the poverty trap that the mentally ill in Ireland were falling into despite the then booming Celtic Tiger economy. The mentally ill were the last in the queue for government money and in the Republic of Ireland, most people with mental health disabilities are worse off than before the boom began. Psychiatry is the Cinderella of the mental health system. 37% of the homeless in Belfast are mentally ill according to in depth research. Due to the nature of the illness, patients often leave hospital with no money or accommodation and Disability Living Allowance forms are unwieldy and hard to fill in. The mentally ill seem to have no way out of the poverty trap, little of them get an education, they can't join the police, army, air force, or navy. Convicted criminals plead insanity to get a lighter sentence. These cases are never out of the news and bring considerable stigma to mental illness in society and the workplace. Having a nervous breakdown can lead to months taken off work and a very harrowing return to work. Many inevitably lose their jobs – indeed, according to BBC research , many employers would rather employ a convicted criminal than a mentally ill person. So the mentally ill remain unemployed and never realise their capabilities in the whole economy.

In 2001, I wrote another article for Fortnight based on a

subject close to my heart – Third Level Education and mental health. Again, this is another area where there is a paucity of knowledge on access to education for the mentally ill, but we do have access to some research. For example, most people diagnosed with a psychotic illness first become ill in their late teens or early twenties – the time when they should be doing GCSEs, A Levels and degrees. Psychosis poses a major interruption. With no further education, few psychiatric survivors gain employment and the majority remain jobless. In certain regions of Northern Ireland, there is no or limited day care facilities for the mentally ill so they have no work routine and as they get older, some have no carer. Therefore it is essential for the mentally ill to be equipped with as much education and life skills as possible.

Stigma, prejudice and fear stop many mental health survivors from taking up educational projects. A prejudicial view from society that they cannot perform the way 'normal' students can is deeply damaging to the morale of the mentally ill. There is also a dearth of knowledge on the benefits of further education to psychiatric survivor. However, some research has surfaced in the USA with studies in Detroit and Canada.

One of the studies found that the process of studying acted as normalisation with many rewards – a chance to step out of the sick role where being a student is seen as normal. It boosted self esteem and confidence as well as a way to learn new tasks.

So given that further education is so empowering to the mentally ill, how do mental health survivors avail themselves of such an opportunity? MIND UK has used computers and IT as an empowering therapeutic medium. This was achieved through intensive one to one tuition, minimum didactic, maximum self-directed ethos where the user designed their own lessons. Ultimately, the degree to which a given society is civilised is indicated in the manner in which that society treats its most vulnerable people. It is society which places barriers to education for mental health sufferers, and society therefore has a responsibility to re-empower those who it has disenfranchised from the educational experience.

In another article for Fortnight, written in October 2004, I attacked the never ending stream of negative stereotypes of the mad and bad mentally ill. Schizophrenia can be seen as a modern version of the disease leprosy and there is a huge amount of ignorance within the general populace towards schizophrenia. The media has a lot of guilt on its hands with its portrayals of 'schizos' and psychos', particularly in the 1980s. There is no other disease in the Western world which receives such opprobrium than schizophrenia. The stigma is perpetuated by films such as Psycho, Silence of the Lambs and Nightmare on Elm Street where madness was seen as criminal, dangerous and psychopathic. Other less well known films such as Repulsion, Friday the 13th and Single White Female also expound upon the mad and bad 'schizo killer'. In fact, the earliest film to portray a homicidal schizo maniac was The Maniac Cook in 1909 which featured the prototype mentally ill homicidal character. As is the convention in these films, the killer keeps coming back to life. This dehumanises the character and discredits those with mental illness to less than human status.

Stigma against the mentally is especially prevalent in the world of accommodation. In Scotland in the 1970s, a rush of horror broke out among 'normal citizens' about the planning of two psychiatric hospitals. Close consultation with the community enabled the Edinburgh unit to go ahead, but the Glasgow unit was subjected to protracted media ignorance and scaremongering.

The media, in fact, do a very good job at whipping up panic by slandering and demonising the mentally ill. An association between violent behaviour and madness has existed in the public mind for hundreds of years. The media has reflected and propagated this stereotype. One study – Signorelli 1989 – found that 72% of mentally ill characters on television drama are portrayed as violent.

Speaking from my own experience, my reputation for having mental health problems has seen me more than once being denied service at bars and nightclubs, and I know of several mental health survivors who have had very similar experiences. And the sad thing is that this kind of denial and stigma is not confined to bars and nightclubs. Certain churches in my area have refused to accommodate a survivor led support network on their premises. This even has an international dimension – you are not allowed to emigrate if you have mental health problems.

So it seems that the stigma of being mentally ill pervades every area of life from jobs to accommodation. This prejudice is not helped by the media. From films to tabloids, this exacerbation is disastrous for anyone suffering acute mental health problems, and since the statistics say one in four of us will visit the doctor's with a mental health complaint, that's a lot of people indeed.

Away from Fortnight magazine, I had prolific dealings with other newspapers and other forms of media. This was part activism and part accolade for my artistic achievements.

Although I did not go on my first trip to Canada until 2002, I was in the Sunday Life in November 2001, thanks to the generosity of Tom Beare MBE who came forth with a donation after seeing my article in the Sunday Life asking for a suitable donation that would take me to Canada for study leave for my PhD. The article stresses my determination to live a normal quality of life despite my mental illness. One of my professors, Mary Chambers, gave a glowing endorsement of my project – to go over and visit an organisation called OCAB (Ontario Council of Alternative Businesses) which is a survivor led business, with a view to starting up something similar with psychiatric survivors in Northern Ireland.

In March 2003 in the Coleraine Times, I announced my

plans for a second trip to Canada – this time for a Madness and Arts World Festival to be held in Toronto. The article mentions that I was to join 100 other artists from countries as diverse as Denmark, Japan, Cuba and Germany. I explained the objectives of my work at the festival – to hold a workshop with Pascale Reboul on poetry and the creative process – imagery and writing practice. I told the Times that I was especially keen to promote the form of performance poetry. The aim of the festival is to get artists together who all have one thing in common – their work explores mental health issues in one way or another.

In the now defunct Daily Ireland newspaper in 2005, in a piece called Breaking Down the Stigma Poetically, I received a glowing write up about my work with psychiatric survivors and the powerful personal testimony of my performance poetry. I spoke of my upcoming journey to Canada and my goals for the trip which included hosting workshops and demonstrating the strange humour behind the world of psychiatry.

On January 31st 2007 my adventures in New Zealand were documented by the Coleraine Chronicle in an article entitled Mind Games in New Zealand. It described my participation in the 'First Annual Nutters Conference of New Zealand'. I was the Conference's Artist in Residence and in the article I described how I like to call the mentally ill – 'survivors' which I think is empowering. The New Zealanders spoke of the mentally ill as users or consumers which is similarly more empowering.

Chapter Eleven THRIVING NOT SURVIVING

Schizoaffective disorder is a very strange illness. It combines all the 'joys' of bipolar disorder or major depression and mixes it up with the vicissitudes of schizophrenia. It is an intensely personal disorder, and no two experiences of the illness will be the same because everyone suffers from it differently. Generally, the sufferer will have a mood component to their illness – experiencing manic or depressed mood as well as suffering from psychotic symptoms such as paranoia, voices, delusions and other schizophrenia-type symptoms. Strangely, given the juxtaposition of schizophrenia and bipolar disorder, Schizoaffective disorder actually has a worse outcome than Bipolar disorder, but a better outcome than schizophrenia. The illness is considered part of the Schizophrenia spectrum along with schizotypal disorder and the lifetime prevalence is between 0.5-0.8 % of the population. No one cause of the illness has been identified but it is thought that genetics, environment, neurobiology etc. may play a part.

People with schizoaffective disorder are likely to have co-morbid disorders such as anxiety and substance abuse disorder. There is also the likelihood of long term social problems such as unemployment, poverty and homelessness. Late adolescence and early adulthood are the most common times of onset. It is an extremely difficult illness to diagnose as it may present as bipolar with psychosis or major depression with psychosis or even plain old schizophrenia. To qualify for a diagnosis, psychosis must be seen in the patient for at least two weeks without major mood disturbances. Untreated, the schizoaffective patient may experience delusions – they may feel watched, monitored or persecuted, or just generally feel a great deal of paranoia. Hallucinations are common too – involving all five senses – hearing voices, strange sensations. There will be a decline in functioning – at school or in personal relationships.

Treatment is usually through a combination of Antipsychotics (Olanzapine, Risperidone, Seroquel) and mood stabilisers (Depakote/Lithium).

I would like to finish the book off by giving an account of not just how I survived, but how I thrived during my two degrees, my travels, my artistic life, my singing career, my media activism and my lecturing career. My main recourse to sanity was through writing poetry and singing. I won the Gay Pride Karaoke competition in July 2008. I believe that artistic expression is vital in the recovery from Schizoaffective disorder and I would urge any sufferer to pursue this route even if it is something as simple as knitting or crocheting, or even baking a cake or preparing a nice meal. This is not just my opinion, there have been several studies produced that have extolled the virtue of creative expression for the mentally ill; ask any Occupational Therapist and they will say this is true. A close friend of mine is also schizoaffective and when she was in hospital for a long stint, she discovered the delights of jewellery making in Occupational Health. She now makes her own jewellery and sells it through local shops, bringing her both money and creative satisfaction. She is now even teaching jewellery making to ladies with disabilities.

I also recommend the art of yoga and relaxation. These both lower the blood pressure and are good for calming the schizoaffective mind, particularly if there is any hypomanic or manic symptoms. My recovery was greatly aided by my pets. I am a cat lover and I have a female spayed cat called Rumpuss who is a constant source of joy and affection to me. It is especially good for people who live on their own to have a pet. Dogs are equally good but require more attention – for example – what do you do when you are in the hospital and you have a dog? Getting around these sorts of issues can be tricky. But I believe that even having a goldfish is therapeutic. However, if you can manage to keep a dog, they are a great source of exercise (through daily walking) which is excellent for the mind and also the body.

Through the years, I have made a habit of walking regularly and also going swimming frequently. Exercise releases serotonin which is a feel good chemical in the brain and the exercise keeps the weight at bay. Unfortunately, as a schizoaffective patient, one is likely to be prescribed antipsychotics as part of the treatment regime. These powerful drugs can inflate your appetite quite considerably and one may end up with dramatic weight gain. Walking is a simple, free and effective form of exercise that will help with the weight gain. Swimming is absolutely brilliant for maintaining a healthy weight if you can keep it up regularly. And both forms of exercise will make you feel good.

The following are a few more tips of things that may help you to thrive, not survive:

- Being in nature and the countryside – whether it is the beach or rural settings, the great outdoors is very soothing for mental health issues. You may like to take up a hobby like bird watching or you might like to go for drives in pleasant surroundings.

- Regulating your diet so that it is healthy and combats the weight gain from antipsychotics will do wonders for your self esteem and your well being.

- Take your medicine regularly as prescribed by your psychiatrist. Going off psychiatric medicine unassisted for any reason can be extremely dangerous.

- Keep a diary to track your moods or levels of psychosis and what triggered it. That way you will get to know your weak spots and what sets you off.

- Try alternative therapies such as Reiki, Aromatherapy and Reflexology. At the very least, they are highly relaxing.

- Plan a daily outing for yourself – don't stay

cloistered in your home, even if it is to go to a friend's house for a chat.

- If you are short on cash, try going to car boot sales and second hand shops to find a bargain. This will give you a feeling of achievement.

- There may be centres for the disabled that you can join and learn arts such as clay, wax working, painting, woodwork, and sewing. It is a great way to meet people.

- Smile, even though you may not feel like it.

- Volunteering is a great way to help other people and also help your self by getting a reference and a set of new skills if you are returning to the work place.

- And finally, candles are extremely relaxing and of course, you can buy them in any scent that is pleasant to you. Just remember to blow them out if you leave the room or go to bed!

Schizo As It Was

Lightning Source UK Ltd.
Milton Keynes UK
UKOW051145280312

189753UK00001B/2/P